Pathophysiology Case Studies

Pathophysiology
Case Studies

Sharon L. Sims, R.N., Ph.D.
Assistant Professor
University of Utah
College of Nursing
Salt Lake City, UT

Donna L. Boland, R.N., Ph.D.
Assistant Professor and
Associate Dean, Undergraduate Programs
Brigham Young University
College of Nursing
Provo, UT

The C. V. Mosby Company

St. Louis • Baltimore • Philadelphia • Toronto   1990

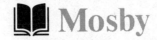

Editor: William Grayson Brottmiller
Senior developmental editor: Sally Adkisson
Project manager: Lin A. Dempsey
Book design: Susan Lane

Printed in the United States of America

The C. V. Mosby Company
11830 Westline Industrial Drive, St. Louis, Missouri 63146

Library of Congress Cataloging-in-Publication Data

Sims, Sharon L.
    Pathophysiology case studies / Sharon L. Sims, Donna L. Boland.
        p.   cm.
    ISBN 0-8016-6223-0
        1. Physiology, Pathological—Case studies.   2. Nursing.
I. Boland, Donna L. II. Title.
[DNLM: 1. Nursing Process–case studies.   2. Nursing Process
problems.   WY 18 S614p]
RB113.S53   1990
616.07'1—dc20
DNLM/DLC
for Library of Congress
                                                                    90-6092
                                                                    CIP

GW/P/P 9 8 7 6 5 4 3 2 1

Contributors

Grace Blodgett, RN, MSN, MBA
Director, Medical Services
Holy Cross Hospital
Salt Lake City, Utah
(AIDS)

Donna Boland, RN, PhD
Assistant Professor
College of Nursing
Brigham Young University
Provo, Utah
(Breast Cancer)

Theresa Brandt, RN, BS
Staff Nurse (formerly)
Surgical Intensive Care Unit
University Hospital
Salt Lake City, Utah
(Surgical ileus)

Karen Brown, RN, PhD, OCN
College of Nursing
University of Utah
Salt Lake City, Utah
(Lung Cancer)

Sherry Brown, RN, MS, CCRN
Clinical Specialist
Surgical Intensive Care Unit
VA Medical Center
Salt Lake City, Utah
(Bacterial meningitis, chronic renal failure, cardiomyopathy)

Shannon Burton, RN, MS
Clinical Assistant Professor
College of Nursing
University of Utah
Salt Lake City, Utah
(Asthma)

Elizabeth Charles, RN, BS
Staff Nurse (formerly)
CCU, MICU
University Hospital
Salt Lake City, Utah
(Acute renal failure)

Pamela F. Cipriano, RN, MN
Director of Nursing Development
Medical University of South Carolina
Charleston, South Carolina
(Hypovolemic shock, alcoholic cirrhosis)

Marilyn Crockett, RN, BS
Head Nurse
Cerebrovascular Unit
University Hospital
Salt Lake City, Utah
(Cerebrovascular Accident)

Janet Egbert-Hansen, RN, MN, CCRN
Instructor
College of Nursing
Brigham Young University
Provo, Utah
(Disseminated Intravascular Coagulation)

Jill Fuller, RN, MS
Assistant Professor
College of Nursing
Minot State University
Minot, North Dakota
(Wound Healing)

Sandra W. Haak, RN, MS
Clinical Assistant Professor
Doctoral Student
College of Nursing
University of Utah
Salt Lake City, Utah
(Hypertension, Myocardial infarction)

Elizabeth Harald, RN, MS
Clinical Assistant Professor
College of Nursing
University of Utah
Salt Lake City, Utah
(Peptic ulcer disease)

Katharine Hoare, RN, DNSC
Assistant Director of Nursing
Nursing Systems
Quality Assurance and Research
Santa Clara Valley Medical Center
San Jose, California
(Degenerative joint disease, rheumatoid arthritis)

Marion Jensen, RN, MS
Associate Professor
College of Nursing
Brigham Young University
Provo, Utah
(Cushing syndrome)

Mary Ann Lambert, RN, MSN
Head Nurse
Neuroscience and Neurological Critical Care Units
University Hospital
Salt Lake City, Utah
(Spinal Cord Injury)

Mary Ann Laubacher, RN, MS, GNP
VA Medical Center
Nashville, Tennessee
(Alzheimer's)

Patti Ludwig-Beymer, RN, Ph.D
Systems Coordinator
Elmhurst College
Deicke Center for Nursing Education
Elmhurst, Illinois
(Diabetes)

Delores Manning, RN, MS
Clinical Specialist (formerly)
NBICU
University Hospital
Salt Lake City, Utah
(Gastroenteritis with dehydration)

Pamela Parker-Cohen, RN, MS, FNPC
Medical Student
Thomas Jefferson Medical College
Philadelphia, Pennsylvania
(Iron-deficiency anemia, urolithiasis, hemophilia A)

Marjorie Peck, RN, PhD
Assistant Administrator, Nursing Services
Alta View, Cottonwood, and LDS Hospitals
Salt Lake City, Utah
(Cystic Fibrosis)

Laurie Rohland, RN, BS
Staff Nurse (formerly)
CCU/MICU
University Hospital
Salt Lake City, Utah
(Emphysema)

Sherrill Scheinblum, RN, MS
Clinical Assistant Professor
University of Utah College of Nursing
(Trisomy 21)

Sharon L. Sims, RN, PhD, PNP
Assistant Professor
College of Nursing
University of Utah
Salt Lake City, Utah
(Ventricular septal defect, hyperthyroidism)

Carolyn Walker, RN, PhD
Assistant Professor
School of Nursing
San Diego State University
San Diego, California
(Acute Lymphocytic Leukemia)

Mary Weissman, RN, BS
Staff Nurse
Intermountain Critical Care Nurses
Salt Lake City, Utah
(Burns)

Pamela Weldele, RN, MS, GNC
Coordinator, Geriatric and Extended Care
Salt Lake Regional Medical Education Center
VA Medical Center
Salt Lake City, Utah
(Bronchopneumonia in the elderly)

Preface

This *Pathophysiology Casebook* was designed to provide a link between theory and practice.

Increasingly, nursing educators have recognized the need for students and practitioners to better understand the underlying disease processes and mechanisms—the pathophysiology—present in the patients they treat. Understanding disease processes promotes better decision making in planning and implementing the care of patients. Assessment data take on greater meaning. Diagnostic statements can be formulated more precisely. Interventions can be more carefully chosen and more effectively implemented. And outcome criteria can be made more specific.

This book cannot substitute for an authoritative textbook on pathophysiology. It can, however, help students and practitioners learn to apply the principles of physiology and human disease to the care of specific patients. In this book, 35 case studies were developed in a single format by nurse experts who specialize in the areas they write about. Introductions are provided that state the specific concepts used in the case study, as well as relevant terminology. Detailed data are presented to provide a lifelike composite of specific patients, including a brief history, clinical manifestations, and a summary of treatment.

The strength of the book lies in the extensive study questions that follow the cases. These test the reader's knowledge of the pathological principles while relating them to an actual individual. Rationales for the correct answers appear in the back of the book. These are so detailed that they serve to extend content covered in textbooks. Ordinarily, a summary is included that explains the outcome of the disease process in the context of the treatment rendered.

Great care has been taken to ensure that all the case studies are presented at a similar level of detail, and that the format is held consistent. The *Pathophysiology Casebook* was originally conceived as an ancillary to accompany a general textbook, *Pathophysiology: The Biologic Basic for Disease in Adults and Children*, by Kathryn L. McCance and Sue E. Huether. In fact, the information included in the case studies receives excellent coverage in the McCance-Huether book. However, the case studies can support the teaching of pathophysiology in courses utilizing any authoritative textbook on pathophysiology or even medical-surgical nursing. Of course, the *Pathophysiology Casebook* can be used by itself as an effective, lifelike review of concepts learned previously.

Sharon L. Sims

Donna L. Boland

Contents

CASE HISTORIES AND STUDY QUESTIONS

CASE STUDY 1   Trisomy 21/Down Syndrome, 3

2   Wound Healing, 6

3   Acquired Immune Deficiency Syndrome (AIDS), 9

4   Breast Cancer, 13

5   Lung Cancer, 17

6   Senile Dementia of the Alzheimer Type (SDAT), 20

7   Spinal Cord Injury, 23

8   Cerebral Vascular Accident (CVA), 26

9   Bacterial Meningitis, 29

10   Hyperthyroidism: Graves Disease, 33

11   Diabetes Mellitus (DM), 36

12   Cushing Syndrome, 39

13   Iron Deficiency Anemia, 41

14   Acute Lymphocytic Leukemia (ALL), 44

15   Disseminated Intravascular Coagulation (DIC) Caused by Septicemia, 47

16   Hemophilia A, 50

17   Hypertension Leading to Congestive Heart Failure (CHF), 54

18   Myocardial Infarction (MI) Caused by Coronary Artery Occlusion, 58

19   Cardiomyopathy, 61

20   Hypovolemic Shock, 64

21   Ventricular Septal Defect (VSD), 67

22   Emphysema, 70

23   Bronchopneumonia in the Elderly, 73

24   Cystic Fibrosis (CF), 76

25   Asthma, 79

26   Urolithiasis, 82

27   Acute Renal Failure, 85

28   Chronic Renal Failure, 88

29   Surgical Ileus, 91

30   Peptic Ulcer Disease, 94

31   Alcoholic Cirrhosis, 97

32   Gastroenteritis with Dehydration, 99

33   Degenerative Joint Disease, 102

34   Rheumatoid Arthritis, 104

35   Burns, 106

ANSWERS WITH RATIONALES

ANSWERS FOR CASE STUDY 1   Trisomy 21/Down Syndrome, 113

2   Wound Healing, 116

3   Acquired Immune Deficiency Syndrome (AIDS), 119

4   Breast Cancer, 121

5   Lung Cancer, 124

6   Senile Dementia of the Alzheimer Type (SDAT), 126

7   Spinal Cord Injury, 129

8   Cerebral Vascular Accident (CVA), 132

9   Bacterial Meningitis, 134

10   Hyperthyroidism: Graves Disease, 138

11   Diabetes Mellitus (DM), 141

12   Cushing Syndrome, 144

13   Iron Deficiency Anemia, 146

14   Acute Lymphocytic Leukemia (ALL), 150

15   Disseminated Intravascular Coagulation (DIC) Caused by Septicemia, 153

16   Hemophilia A, 155

17   Hypertension Leading to Congestive Heart Failure (CHF), 159

18   Myocardial Infarction (MI) Caused by Coronary Artery Occlusion, 161

19   Cardiomyopathy, 164

20   Hypovolemic Shock, 167

21   Ventricular Septal Defect (VSD), 169

22   Emphysema, 171

23   Bronchopneumonia in the Elderly, 173

24   Cystic Fibrosis (CF), 175

25 Asthma, 177

26 Urolithiasis, 179

27 Acute Renal Failure, 182

28 Chronic Renal Failure, 185

29 Surgical Ileus, 189

30 Peptic Ulcer Disease 191

31 Alcoholic Cirrhosis, 193

32 Gastroenteritis with Dehydration, 195

33 Degenerative Joint Disease, 198

34 Rheumatoid Arthritis, 200

35 Burns, 202

Pathophysiology Case Studies

CASE HISTORIES AND STUDY QUESTIONS

1 Trisomy 21/Down syndrome

This case study will incorporate the following concepts:
 1. Embryonic development
 2. Disruption in normal fetal genetic development
 3. Mechanisms associated with genetic development
 4. Down syndrome
 5. Genetic counseling

CASE HISTORY

Mrs. H. is a 45-year-old primipara who was admitted to the labor and delivery unit. She was accompanied by her 48-year-old husband. She walked into the labor room unassisted and in apparent good health. This first delivery is the culmination of an uneventful pregnancy. Mrs. H. did have severe episodes of morning sickness during her first trimester but has had no further complications. Admitting blood pressure was 135/78; maternal pulse was 80; and fetal heart rate was 140 beats/min. Six hours after admission, Mrs. H. delivered a 7-pound, 8-ounce baby boy.

STUDY QUESTIONS

1. The delivery room nurse immediately noticed that the baby had low-set ears, a low flat nasal bridge, a protruding tongue, and wide epicanthal folds. These characteristics lead the nurse to suspect:
   a. that the baby had experienced facial trauma because of a left-mentoanterior presentation
   b. that the episodes of morning sickness had created a metabolic disturbance interfering with normal cellular development
   c. that these characteristics are most properly related to some sort of chromosomal defect
   d. that trauma to the cord had occurred, creating these deformities

2. When Mrs. H. returns to her room the baby is brought to her for his feeding. As Mrs. H. feeds the baby she is able to examine him closely. She notices that his eyes are different and appear slanted and, as she inspects his hands, she finds he has creases extending the full width of his palms. Even though the physician has informed them that their infant has trisomy 21, during her questions to the nurse regarding her findings it becomes apparent that she does not fully understand the physical features of this condition. Which of the following is true of the baby's appearance?
   a. These two findings are called epicanthal folds and simian creases, respectively; these findings are seen in approximately 50% of all babies born with trisomy 21
   b. Although epicanthal folds and simian creases are characteristic of trisomy 21, they also appear in a large percentage of the normal population
   c. These two features are characteristic of trisomy 21, which is the result of a genetic defect that happened during the third trimester of fetal development
   d. Both the epicanthal folds and the simian creases will become less apparent as the child grows and develops along a normal pattern

3. Although a majority of chromosomal aberrations are sporadic, they can, on occasion, be directly inherited. The genetic basis for the baby's aberration will be identified by:
   a. thoroughly analyzing his phenotype
   b. establishing the presence of Barr bodies
   c. analyzing the chromosomal formation of his white blood cells
   d. establishing the chromosomal patterns in both parents

4. From your knowledge of genetic development, you know that nondisjunction is the chromosome aberration that is most likely responsible for the infant's condition. Chromosomal nondisjunction is best described as:
   a. failure of the centromeres to separate during the metaphase of mitosis
   b. failure of the parent cell to form two new nuclei during the telophase of mitosis
   c. a mixup in the placement of the genes on the chromosomes during meiosis
   d. failure of two chromosomes to separate during the first meiotic phase of cellular division

5. Mr. and Mrs. H., in struggling to understand what happened to their baby, have asked you for an explanation of how this could have happened to them. Of the following statements which one best explains what happened genetically?
   a. Down syndrome is a genetically inherited disease caused when both parents are carriers
   b. Trisomy 21 is a sex-linked disease that occurs when the sex gametes fail to separate during cellular division
   c. Down syndrome occurs when the chromosomes fail to divide properly, usually as a result of multiple factors
   d. Down syndrome is the result of a chromosome missing from the normal cellular karyotype

6. During the first 24 hours after birth, the nurses in the nursery are carefully watching the baby for abdominal distention. They note that he has passed no stool since birth. Which of the following has to be considered in the nursing assessment?
    a. This is a common pattern among the majority of newborns
    b. Metabolic and enzyme functions are frequently altered in Down syndrome babies
    c. Down syndrome babies are poor feeders and, as a result, have a sluggish gastrointestinal system
    d. The baby is showing early signs of allergies to his formula

7. Mr. and Mrs. H. are concerned about the physical problems their son may have. Which of the following is the most accurate statement the nurse could make?
    a. Babies with Down syndrome have functional abnormalities at about the same rate as normal babies
    b. Functional abnormalities in Down syndrome are randomly distributed; therefore, it is difficult to predict the risks for the baby
    c. The only known abnormalities associated with Down syndrome are heart defects and intestinal atresia
    d. Babies with Down syndrome often have cardiac anomalies, respiratory infections, kidney problems, and tracheoesophageal fistulae

8. The parents are also concerned about their son's degree of mental retardation. What can the nurse tell them?
    a. Every child with Down syndrome has some degree of mental retardation but most have IQs within the "trainable" range
    b. The average IQ for a child with Down syndrome is 30
    c. Most children with Down syndrome are only minimally retarded
    d. Most children with Down syndrome are severely retarded, and institutionalization is usually the best treatment option

2 Wound Healing

This case study will incorporate the following concepts:
1. *Dysfunctional wound healing*
2. *Healing by primary intention*
3. *Principles of wound care*

CASE HISTORY

Mrs. P. is a 65-year-old woman with a history of type I diabetes mellitus. Although insulin-dependent for many years, she has enjoyed relatively good health, which she attributes to her regular self-administration of insulin. She is moderately overweight and was diagnosed as hypertensive 10 years ago. Her hypertension has been under control since she was placed on a thiazide diuretic.

Past History

Mrs. P. was planning to drive to the market one morning and discovered that her automobile would not start. After calling a family member to fix her car, she decided to walk the two blocks to the market. Rather than change into her usual walking shoes, she wore the more fashionable new shoes she had originally put on that morning. After her return home, Mrs. P. removed her shoes and noted a small blister on the bottom of her left heel. She felt no discomfort associated with this blister; in fact, she may not have noticed its initial appearance if she had not inspected her feet.

The following day Mrs. P. was alarmed to note that the small blister had become a large, open wound resembling a crater that was bluish black in color. For the next 3 days, Mrs. P. carefully cleansed her heel wound and covered it with sterile gauze. Noting that the wound looked progressively worse, she reported to her family physician on the fourth day after injury.

Current Status

Mrs. P.'s heel wound is 5 cm in diameter, and the wound bed contains necrotic tissue. There is no evidence of angiogenesis or granulation tissue formation. Mrs. P. has evidence of impaired circulation to her legs, and pedal and posterior tibial pulses are not palpable bilaterally. Both feet are cool to touch and her toes are slightly cyanotic. She has a mild temperature elevation (37.9° C) and her serum glucose is 360 mg/dl.

Wound and blood cultures were obtained. Her complete blood count revealed a leukocytosis. Mrs. P. was admitted to the hospital, placed on bedrest, and started on broad-spectrum antibiotic therapy while waiting culture and sensitivity reports. The wound was packed with saline-soaked kerlix gauze to facilitate debridement of necrotic tissue. Serum glucose levels were determined every 4 hours, and regular insulin was administered according to a sliding scale. The wound culture reports were eventually completed and revealed a wound grossly contaminated with many species of gram-negative bacteria. Blood culture reports were negative. The wound showed no signs of healing after several days of treatment. A decision was made to perform a below-the-knee amputation to prevent a fatal systemic infection.

STUDY QUESTIONS

1. Which of the following processes of normal wound healing was most impaired by Mrs. P.'s diabetic condition?
   a. Inflammation
   b. Collagen metabolism
   c. Epithelialization
   d. Contraction

2. The initial treatment of Mrs. P.'s wound represented an attempt to promote healing by:
   a. primary intention
   b. secondary intention
   c. third intention

Mrs. P. undergoes surgery for a left below-the-knee amputation. The amputation stump is closed by means of a skin flap. A long, sutured midline incision is present. The incision is covered with petrolatum gauze and soft cotton padding. The entire stump is then wrapped with an elastic compression bandage. A drain is placed in the wound bed at the time of surgery. The stump is to be unwrapped and inspected twice a day, and a new dressing is then applied, using sterile technique. Serum glucose continues to be closely monitored as it was preoperatively. Mrs. P. is started on parenteral feedings and the usual postoperative practice of coughing and deep breathing exercises is initiated.

On the third postoperative day, the wound is unwrapped for a dressing change. The petrolatum gauze pulls away readily from the incision line and is saturated with mucopurulent drainage. The incision line is reddened and painful when palpated with a gloved hand. The drain is still intact with return of only a scant amount of serosanguineous drainage. Mrs. P.'s temperature is 38.2° C. White blood cell count is elevated. Arterial Po_2 is 68 mm Hg. Mrs. P. is depressed and withdrawn.

3. Signs and symptoms of wound infection include all of the following except:
   a. pain
   b. hypoxemia
   c. purulent discharge
   d. edema

4. The purpose of the drain in the wound is to:
   a. serve as an escape route for mucopurulent drainage should an infection develop
   b. provide continuous pressure needed for proper orientation of collagen molecules
   c. decrease the wound dead space that may occur with accumulation of blood and fluid
   d. prevent the development of flexion contractures

5. Additional debriding is indicated along the suture line since there is mucopurulent drainage present. The most appropriate method of debridement would be:
   a. application of wet to dry dressings
   b. application of antiseptic gauze (betadine)
   c. high-pressure pulsatile irrigations
   d. hydrogen peroxide-soaked dressings

6. Of the following, which is the most essential nutrient during this phase of Mrs. P.'s recovery?
   a. vitamin C
   b. calcium
   c. glucose
   d. iron

3 Acquired Immune Deficiency Syndrome (AIDS)

This case study will incorporate the following concepts:
  1. Etiology of AIDS
  2. Risk associated behaviors
  3. Evaluation of human immune deficiency virus (HIV) infected status
  4. Antiviral/antimicrobial agents
  5. Supportive care
  6. Disease progression and life expectancy of AIDS patients

CASE HISTORY

D.L., a 32-year-old Caucasian male, was admitted to the hospital with symptoms of a depressed immune system, including oral and groin candidiasis (thrush) and a herpes virus infection. This is his fourth admission in less than 2 years.

Past History

D.L. is a homosexual and has engaged in anal and oral intercourse since the age of 20. He was treated for condylomata (venereal warts) approximately 3 years ago, with resolution. In October 1988 he presented with oral and groin candidiasis and perianal lesions, which on culture revealed a herpes infection. His past sexual behavior and current viral infections warranted antibody testing (enzyme linked immunosorbent assay [ELISA] and western blot,) which yielded positive findings. He commenced a treatment protocol that included zidovudine (azathioprine [AZT] Retrovir), tuberculous prophylaxis, and clotrimazole (Mycelex Troches).

D.L. has had four inpatient admissions and three outpatient transfusion admissions between November 1988 and December 1989. In November 1988, he presented to the clinic complaining of a loss of appetite resulting in a 10-pound weight loss over a 2-week period, a nonproductive cough, some shortness of breath, and a perianal lesion. He tested HIV-positive. Symptoms were severe enough to warrant hospital admission.

Admitting chest roentgenogram revealed diffuse infiltrates compatible with *Pneumocystis carinii* pneumonia (PCP) and *Mycobacterium avium intercellulare* (MAI). An induced sputum demonstrated the presence of the pneumocystis microorganism, and a skin lesion scraping grew herpes and cytomegalovirus (CMV). He commenced oral trimethoprim-sulfamethoxazole (Septa Bactrim), in response to which he developed an allergic rash and a fever of 102° F. A course of intravenous pentamidine isethionate controlled the symptoms of PCP and he was discharged to receive prophylactic, inhaled pentamidine isethionate every 2 weeks. A topical application of acyclovir and zinc oxide was instituted for the perianal ulceration. He was found to be anemic in April 1989 (hematocrit 22.3 ml; hemoglobin 7.8 g) and was transfused with 2 units of blood as an outpatient.

Two months later, D.L. presented to the emergency room complaining of severe abdominal pain accompanied by diarrhea and bloody stools for the last 2 weeks. He had lost 25 pounds. He also complained of transient pain and numbness of his hands and feet that warranted medication. A spinal tap was performed; the result was negative for herpes, CMV, and Cryptococcus. A gastrointestinal series and stool culture demonstrated the mycobacterial microorganism. He was transfused with 4 units of blood, received loperamide hydrochloride (Imodium and Lomotil) for the diarrhea, and was discharged home.

D.L. was again admitted in July 1989. He was emaciated and had atrophy of both hands and feet, foot drop, moderate shortness of breath, and situational depression. A bone marrow aspiration revealed severe compromise. D.L.'s poor prognosis was discussed with him, and he requested not to be resuscitated. He inadvertently, or deliberately, took 10 triazolam (Halcion) pills but on psychiatric evaluation was not considered to be suicidal. His AZT was discontinued in view of his bone marrow depression. His respiratory condition deteriorated and a bronchoscopy was performed. Examination revealed the presence of severe infiltrates with PCP and a resultant arterial saturation level of 32% and a carbon dioxide level of 42% that warranted ventilatory support, with the understanding that no cardiac compression be instituted if arrest occurred. Tube feedings (Osmolite) were started and ventilatory support continued for 3 days, during which time he received intravenous pentamidine isethionate and 4 units of blood. His condition improved and he was extubated. One week after admission he commenced physical therapy for foot drop and progressive ambulation. He made significant progress and was discharged home with oxygen, several types of medication, and psychiatric and continuity of care (bereavement, spiritual, financial) support.

D.L.'s physical and psychiatric condition continued to worsen over the next few months. He required two additional blood transfusions and a third hospitalization.

Current Status

In December 1989, D.L. was admitted to the hospital in an extremely confused state. His temperature was 103° F. Chest roentgenogram revealed severe pulmonary infiltrations, and MAI and herpes infected lesions were found to be resistant to antibiotic therapy. In addition, D. was suffering from severe bone marrow depression, severe diarrhea, vomiting, and Kaposi's sarcoma of the skin. Antiemetics, steroids, analgesics, and antidiarrhetic drug therapies were implemented as terminal comfort measures. D. expired 3 days later.

1. In helping D.L. deal with his diagnosis, the nurse needs to know that AIDS manifests as reduced resistance to opportunistic infections and malignancies caused by:
   a. an acquired deficiency of isoimmunity
   b. an exaggerated immune response to counteract a T-cell deficiency
   c. impaired functioning of one or more components of the immune/inflammatory response
   d. deficiency of antigen (HIV) recognition

2. The T_4 helper cell to T_8 suppressor cell ratio is normally about 2:1. This ratio in D.L. was severely reduced because:
   a. Bone marrow depression reduces hemoglobin and hematocrit levels
   b. The HIV virus infects and kills the host T_4 cells decreasing their numbers
   c. The T_8 suppressor cells are stimulated by the HIV virus, and their numbers increase
   d. γ-Interferon is reduced, thereby reducing cytotoxic T_8 suppressor cell activity

3. The main reason an AIDS vaccine does not currently exist for high-risk individuals like D.L. is that:
   a. Research on vaccines is extremely expensive and time-consuming
   b. It is ethically unacceptable to inject humans with attenuated vaccines
   c. It is difficult to obtain volunteers for needed research trials
   d. HIV is variable and often has a prolonged period of dormancy.

4. PCP (a protozoon), normally nonpathogenic, caused severe respiratory problems for D.L. caused by:
   a. the bacterial invasion of PCP into his lungs
   b. pleural effusion caused by the proliferation of the PCP
   c. the filling of the alveoli with eosinophilic exudate and PCP
   d. other superimposed infections masked by his medication

5. The severity of D.L.'s diarrhea was most probably caused by:
   a. reactivation of previously present microorganisms
   b. HIV-induced malabsorption
   c. antibiotic therapy
   d. severe depression and anxiety

6. D.L.'s confusion and distal peripheral neuropathy, in light of negative serological findings, was most likely caused by:
   a. primary or secondary central nervous system lymphoma
   b. Toxoplasma, a protozoon infecting the central nervous system
   c. disturbance in normal brain patterns from a pharmacokinetic disruption in the drug therapy
   d. presence of HIV virus in peripheral nerves and the central nervous system

7. The nurse needs to monitor D.L. continually for which frequently observed neurological symptomatic triad?
   a. Kaposi's sarcoma, PCP, and cryptococcal meningitis
   b. cognitive, motor, and behavioral changes
   c. seizures, paresthesias, and dysthesias
   d. seizures, depression, and paresthesias

8. D.L.'s repeated episodes with MAI and herpes and limited response to medications
   indicated:
   a. inability to comply with treatment protocols
   b. loss of antibiotic therapy effectiveness after repeated treatment
   c. inability to eradicate infections associated with advanced stages of AIDS
   d. inability to maintain therapeutic levels of medication

4 Breast Cancer

This case study will incorporate the following concepts:
  1. Risk factors associated with breast cancer
  2. Properties of cancer cells, including differentiation, proliferation, and spread
  3. Morbidity and mortality

CASE HISTORY

Mrs. C. is a 47-year-old Caucasian female who has been admitted to the general surgical floor with a lump in her right breast.

Past History

Mrs. C. has generally enjoyed good health up to this admission. She neither smokes nor drinks and follows a daily exercise regimen. Approximately 2 months ago Mrs. C.'s husband noticed a small lump in her right breast. She gave this finding little attention, assuming that the lump was like the many others that she tends to experience around her menses. The lump, however, failed to follow the general pattern of resolution and Mrs. C. became concerned when it seemed to grow bigger. Mrs. C. is married and the mother of two children, one 8 and the other 6. Mrs. C. took birth control pills for 5 years after the birth of her second child. Last year she chose to discontinue use of these and turned to an alternative method of birth control. Mrs. C. is the only child born to her parents late in their life. Her father is alive and well, but her mother died of breast cancer 5 years ago. A further family history reveals that there is a strong history of both heart disease and cancer on both sides of Mrs. C.'s family.

Current Status

On examination a 2- to 3-cm mass was palpated in the upper quadrant of her right breast. This mass felt firm, was fixed to the chest wall, and was tender to the touch. The remaining breast skin was normal in appearance with no discoloration or retraction of the skin. The nipple was neither inverted nor draining. One node, approximately the size of a pea, was palpated under the right axilla. Palpation of the left breast revealed two 1- to 2-cm soft, movable masses. Mrs. C. said that she noticed these lumps in her left breast 2 weeks ago. She states that the lumps in her left breast became palpable and bothersome about 12 days from the start of menstruation. At present she is about 5 days from this start date. A reproductive history disclosed that the onset of menses occurred at the age of 10. There is no history of dysmenorrhea associated with her periods, although she states that her breasts become tender and "lumpy" a week or two before her period. She has had no pregnancies that were delivered by caesarean section. Her one and only Papanicolaou smear was done 2 years ago and produced a normal result. The remainder of the examination findings were unremarkable.

Mammography confirmed the presence of a 3-cm mass in the upper quadrant of the right breast. It was also noted that three 1.5 cm masses were visible in the left breast. The result of a bone scan was negative, as were those of a number of other diagnostic procedures.

STUDY QUESTIONS

1. Mrs. C. is considered to be at increased risk for developing breast cancer. Which of the following factors is most positively related to this high-risk profile?
   a. history of breast cancer in family members
   b. history of cystic breast disease
   c. early onset of menarche
   d. trauma related to the birth of her children

2. Which of the following best explains the existence of an enlarged right axillary lymph node in Mrs. C.?
   a. The lymph node is the result of an inflammatory reaction that normally occurs with the onset of her current menses
   b. The existence of the node is the result of an increased strain on the lymphatic system as a result of cellular degeneration
   c. The lymph node exists to provide nutrients to the rapidly growing cancer cells
   d. The lymph node is the result of cancer cells' spreading to different tissues within the body

3. Although Mrs. C. complained that the lumps noted in both breasts were tender, the lump in the right breast felt different from those in the left breast. How would you explain this difference?
   a. The mass in the right breast has been present for a longer period of time than those in the left breast
   b. The mass in the right breast is the result of a different pattern of cellular proliferation than that taking place in the left
   c. The mass in the right breast is encapsulated, whereas the masses in the left breast have already started to metastasize to surrounding tissue
   d. The mass in the right breast is experiencing an increase in the flow of interstitial fluid caused by the phagocytosis process

Mrs. C. was taken to surgery 3 days later, and a modified radical mastectomy was performed. A histological examination allowed the pathologist to classify the tumor by using the tumor/nodes/metastasis (TNM) staging system. An estrogen receptor assay was also done on the removed tissue; it confirmed that Mrs. C.'s tumor was estrogen-dependent. She returned to her room with a Hemovac in place. Her dressing was dry and intact. She was able to turn, cough, and deep breathe on her own. Her temperature remained within normal limits after surgery. Ambulation was started on the second post-operative day.

4. On the third postoperative day, Mrs. C.'s right arm became increasingly edematous and painful. What is the best explanation for the lymphedema presently being experienced?
   a. An electrolyte imbalance is creating an increase in the hydrostatic pressure in the lymphatic system
   b. A postoperative infection has produced the beginnings of an immune response from the T lymphocytes
   c. The lymphatic channels are congested with fat particles that are being displaced from the trauma of surgery
   d. The remaining lymph nodes are inadequate to handle the lymph flow, creating an increase in the hydrostatic pressure

5. Mrs. C.'s tumor was staged at T2a;Nlb;MO using the TNM staging system. Pathological examination of the surgically removed tissue sample placed Mrs. C.'s tumor in category type II. The need to stage and classify tumors is important for which of the following reasons?
   a. Treatment is based on the knowledge of tumor size, extent, and tissue type
   b. Tumor staging is useful for studying a number of researchable factors from survival to treatment response
   c. A consistent classification system provides a way to catalogue individuals with breast tumors for statistical analysis
   d. All of the above

6. As soon as Mrs. C. starts to feel better and is performing most activities of daily living (ADLs) unassisted, her nurse begins educating her on how to care for her affected arm and hand. Although Mrs. C. has always been careful about grooming, she wonders whether all the dos and don'ts given her are necessary. On the basis of your knowledge of breast surgery, which explanation is most appropriate to help Mrs. C. better understand the rationale behind meticulous hand and skin care?
   a. Lymphedema can be aggravated by any kind of trauma to the hand from a cut, a burn, or anything causing prolonged pressure to the area
   b. It is important to keep your hands clean and free of cuts to prevent bacteria from being spread to the surgical site
   c. Involvement of skin care on the affected site will help Mrs. C. psychologically accept the fact that she had a mastectomy
   d. Skin care is critical in decreasing the amount of circulating viruses within the body as cancer cells are easily transported by these viruses

7. At the time of discharge, Mrs. C.'s physician started her on hormonal therapy. The underlying physiological rationale for this treatment is that:
   a. Now that half of the excretory ducts are missing, Mrs. C. will require hormonal replacement
   b. Without estrogen replacement the remaining breast will shrink and become a non-functioning lactating structure
   c. Circulating androgens will easily bind with poorly differentiated cells, preventing spread of these cells
   d. Hormones will bind with the DNA in the nucleus, causing a transcription in the coding that affects cell viability

5 Lung Cancer

This case study will incorporate the following concepts:
1. Etiology of lung cancers
2. Risk factors associated with development of lung cancer
3. Pathophysiology of lung cancers
4. Manifestation of lung cancers
5. Diagnostic procedures utilized in detection of lung cancer
6. Respiratory assessment skills

CASE HISTORY

Mr. G. is a 58-year-old black, blue-collar worker. He has smoked for approximately 45 pack/years. Pack/years are calculated by number of packs/day, times number of years; thus, someone smoking 10 pack/years has smoked 1 pack/day for 10 years or 2 packs/day for 5 years.

Past History

Mr. G.'s family history is negative for lung cancers, though other relatives have been diagnosed with cancer: a maternal aunt with ovarian cancer, a grandmother with breast cancer, and a nephew with Burkitt lymphoma. Mr. G.'s environmental history indicates he worked with asbestos in both construction and shipbuilding during World War II. He lives in a large metropolitan area, approximately half a mile away from a heavily traveled interstate highway.

Current Status

Mr. G. has experienced bothersome dizziness and headaches over the last 2 weeks. On the day of admission, he experienced an episode of blurring vision associated with vertigo and tinnitus. He has also noticed a vague pain or stiffness in his left arm and shoulder and attributes this to "old age creepin' up." His usual morning "smoker's cough" has lengthened to last all day, with increasing frequency of hemoptysis. Mr. G. states he has always been prone to "lung problems" and does not "pay them much mind." When asked whether he experiences dyspnea on exertion, he laughs and replies in the affirmative, adding that this is from his smoking and does not worry him. Mr. G. says he has been in the hospital once or twice for lung problems and was treated medically with "IV and oxygen" for bronchitis and other conditions he cannot recall. Postural nocturnal dyspnea necessitates that he sleep in his reclining chair, propped up with pillows so he is sitting straight up. Lately he has found it necessary to sleep hunched over the kitchen table resting his head and arms on pillows.

Physical examination reveals a middle-aged black male in respiratory distress. Buccal mucosa and nailbeds are dusky, and he cannot complete a sentence without drawing a breath. He exhibits clubbing. He has a positive Romberg's sign, and Rinne's test reveals air conduction greater than bone conduction bilaterally. Pupils are equal, are round, and react sluggishly to light and accommodation. Mr. G.'s respiratory exam reveals an anteroposterior to transverse diameter of 1:1. Expansion is less than 2 cm bilaterally, and diaphragmatic excursion is 1 to 2 cm bilaterally. Mr. G. is using accessory muscles (intercostals) to breathe. Percussion reveals tympany over lung fields with an area of resonance to dullness over the right middle lobe in the midaxillary line at the seventh intercostal space. Tactile fremitus is found to be greater over this area and diminished over the remainder of Mr. G.'s lobes. Decreased breath sounds are evident on auscultation, with vocal fremitus increased over the area of dullness described. A unilateral wheeze on inspiration is evident. Respiratory rate is 24. Cervical and axillary lymph nodes are slightly enlarged, fixed, and nontender. Other physical findings are nonspecific.

Chest roentgenograms, anteroposterior (A-P) and lateral, indicate a mass displacing the left bronchus roughly corresponding to the area of dullness and increased tactile fremitus. Complete blood count is within normal limits except for a borderline low hematocrit. Radioisotope scans indicate positive bone involvement in the left humerus and scapula. Head roentgenogram reveals questionable bilateral displacement of ventricles and areas of shadow. Bronchoscopic histology indicates a small cell carcinoma, also known as oat cell. Bone marrow aspiration and biopsy results indicate marrow involvement.

STUDY QUESTIONS

1. Which of the following most likely accounts for Mr. G.'s headaches?
   a. dyspnea
   b. living and working in a stressful environment
   c. metastatic involvement
   d. muscle tension from painful shoulder and arm

2. Which of the following has probably accounted for Mr. G.'s development of oat cell cancer of the lung?
   a. history of working with asbestos
   b. 45-pack/year history of smoking
   c. living in an urban environment near known carcinogens
   d. all of the above

3. Mr. G. should not be put on oxygen therapy without caution. Why?
    a. Damaged lung tissue will not benefit from increasing oxygen
    b. His symptoms are not caused by lack of oxygen, so it will not help
    c. He might suffer respiratory arrest
    d. He has not been admitted with the same problems that were treated with oxygen in the past

4. Physiologically, Mr. G.'s oat cell carcinoma combined with a long history of smoking results in the clinical manifestations described because of:
    a. destruction of alveoli secondary to abuse (smoking) and disease
    b. chemical agents released from the tumor and metastic sites
    c. hereditary predispositions that have led to clubbing and enlarged A-P chest ratio
    d. tumors partially obstructing the bronchi that result in poor ventilation

5. Note that on auscultation, Mr. G.'s wheezes occur unilaterally on the right. This phenomenon was most likely caused by:
    a. inability of air to reach the alveoli because of thickened bronchi
    b. other respiratory ailments for which Mr. G. was hospitalized earlier
    c. his anxiety's decreasing his ability to expand his lungs fully
    d. a tumor pressing on the bronchi or unilaterally, inhibiting air from entering the lower lobe without turbulence

6. Mr. G.'s therapies for oat cell carcinoma include chemotherapy (Cytoxan) and radiation therapy. These two diverse therapies are similar in which of the following aspects?
    a. Both chemotherapy (Cytoxan) and radiation therapy destroy tumor cells by inhibiting or altering the ability of DNA and RNA to complete mitosis successfully
    b. Chemotherapy and radiation therapy destroy the fastest producing body cells, including hair follicles and gastrointestinal mucosa
    c. Both therapies result in bone marrow suspension that may result in thrombocytopenia (low thrombocyte count)
    d. All of the above

Mr. G. is treated with chemotherapy (Cytoxan) intravenously. He is then sent home and scheduled for outpatient radiation therapy treatments for palliation of bony metastatic pain. He is followed in the clinic and radiation therapy department by his oncologist. Surgery is not deemed helpful because of the extensive involvement at the time of diagnosis. Treatment goals are to palliate the growth and discomfort of the disease and to maintain quality of life for as long as possible. Mr. G. becomes progressively more dyspneic and experiences more pain as the months progress. He dies 8 1/2 months after initial diagnosis.

6 Senile Dementia of the Alzheimer Type (SDAT)

This case study will incorporate the following concepts:
 1. Reversible causes of dementia
 2. Diagnosis of dementia
 3. Etiology of senile dementia of the Alzheimer type
 4. Medication use
 5. Neuropathological changes in SDAT

CASE HISTORY

Mrs. K., a 76-year-old retired bookkeeper, was first seen by her family physician for evaluation of memory loss and personality changes at the insistence of her husband and three children.

Past History

Over the past 2 years, Mr. K. had observed that his wife could not handle simple finances accurately despite her many years of successful employment as a bookkeeper. Memory problems had become apparent to the family and friends but were attributed to absentmindedness. Maintaining Mrs. K.'s social relationships became difficult as she developed problems remembering names, dates, and places.

Initially, Mrs. K. was distressed about her forgetfulness and expressed concern that she was becoming "senile like Aunt Helen." As her memory and cognitive function declined, she denied having any problems. Managing her behavior was often difficult as she became angry and suspicious toward her family, especially her husband.

Current Status

A complete history was taken, and physical examination of Mrs. K. that included a functional ability assessment was performed. A medication history revealed that she had been taking ibuprofen, hydrochlorothiazide, and potassium chloride for management of degenerative joint disease and essential hypertension. A mental status examination was performed, and the following diagnostic studies were ordered: complete blood count, complete serum chemistry assessment, rapid plasma reagin (RPR) test, thyroid function tests, serum B_{12} and folate levels, urinalysis, electrocardiogram, electroencephalogram, and computed tomography (CT) scan of the brain.

STUDY QUESTIONS

1. Mrs. K's examination included diagnostic tests specific for ruling out possible reversible causes of dementia. Results of which diagnostic evaluations and/or tests support a diagnosis of SDAT?
   a. complete blood count and chemistry evaluation
   b. electrocardiogram and CT scan
   c. mental status examination and progressive course of the dementia
   d. past medical history, functional ability, and physical examination

2. Depression, a common problem in older people, is often diagnosed and treated as dementia. How can depression be distinguished from dementia?
   a. Depressed clients often complain of memory problems, whereas demented clients try to conceal memory impairment
   b. The onset of dementia is rapid and obvious, whereas identifying the onset of depression is usually difficult
   c. The demented person has very stable and apathetic behavior patterns, whereas the depressed person has a wide fluctuation of behavior
   d. The depressed person has little or no change in self-image, whereas the demented person has a poor self-image

3. Multiinfarct dementia (MID) has to be ruled out as a possible cause of Mrs. K.'s dementia. MID is associated with:
   a. elevated blood glucose levels and diabetes
   b. hypertension and cardiovascular diseases
   c. alcohol and drug abuse
   d. infections in the central nervous system

Mrs. K. became more confused over the next few years. She had periods of agitation that led to wandering and occasional assaultive behavior. She required assistance with feeding, dressing, and bathing. She had difficulty finding the bathroom and could not remember how to toilet herself. She became increasingly restless and anxious in the evening. In the middle of the night her husband would find her wandering through the house, and he often took an hour or more to persuade her to go back to sleep. Mrs. K. was started on thioridazine.

4. Thioridazine is a major tranquilizer. How is this drug used for the client with SDAT?
   a. It is given in high doses to stimulate the production of dopamine in the brain
   b. It is used in controlled experimental trials for the treatment of dementia
   c. It is only used in small doses to treat depression that can accompany dementia
   d. It is used in small doses to control disruptive and destructive behavior

Eventually Mrs. K.'s care became too difficult for her family to manage at home. She was admitted to a long-term care facility because she could no longer walk, feed herself, or control her bowel and bladder functions. She developed difficulty swallowing and took fluids poorly. Managing urinary tract infections, and constipation and preventing skin breakdown were constant care needs.

5. The degenerative course of SDAT impacts not only mental but physiological function. Individuals with SDAT commonly die of:
   a. renal failure
   b. malnutrition
   c. pneumonia
   d. decubitus ulcers

6. The family requests an autopsy after Mrs. K.'s death. What brain tissue changes would confirm a diagnosis of SDAT?
   a. neurofibrillary tangles and amyloid plaques
   b. multiple areas of infarcted brain tissue throughout the cerebellum
   c. generalized cerebral hypertrophy
   d. vascular insufficiency

7 Spinal Cord Injury

This case study will incorporate the following concepts:
1. *Spinal shock*
2. *Motor and sensory involvement in spinal cord injury*
3. *Phases of return of spinal cord activity*
4. *Autonomic dysreflexia*
5. *Gastrointestinal system effects*
6. *Genitourinary effects*

CASE HISTORY

A.D. is a 19-year-old college student who was rock climbing and fell 30 feet to the ground.

Past History

A.D. is 6 feet 7 inches and very active on his college basketball team. His medical history is relatively negative except for the usual childhood illnesses and minor accidents. On his basketball physical examination before school started, his vital signs were as follows: blood pressure 110/82; heart rate 88; respirations 18.

Current Status

A.D. was picked up at the scene of the accident by paramedics who found him lying in a supine position, unable to move any extremities and complaining of some neck discomfort. He appeared awake, alert, and oriented to his current location, the date and day of the week, and details of the fall. His responses to verbal questioning were appropriate. He complained that he could not feel or move his arms and legs. His pupils were equal and reactive to light. He showed no signs of other injury except for several scrapes on his arms. His vital signs revealed blood pressure of 110/72; heart rate of 86; respirations of 18, unlabored and regular. The paramedics applied a cervical collar, placed him on a back board, immobilized his head, and transported to the medical center by helicopter.

A.D. was found to exhibit no deep tendon reflexes of the extremities in the emergency room. His perception of sensory stimulus ended just above the nipple line of the chest. He had some sensory perception of the arms but was not able to demonstrate any consistent pattern of perception with repeated examinations. He had some ability to tighten the biceps but could not overcome gravity to raise his arms. He was unable to expand his chest wall minimally on midthorax expansion. The remainder of his physical examination revealed blood pressure at 100/60; heart rate 68; respirations 24, somewhat shallow; oral temperature 99.8° F. His color was dusky. His skin was warm and dry to touch. A.D. was asking questions of his physicians during his examination and was quite upset and expressed fear of being paralyzed.

Roentgenograms of the full spine, skull, and chest were ordered. A complete blood panel with arterial gases was drawn. Intravenous lactated Ringer's solution was started and a Foley catheter inserted into the bladder. A nasogastric tube was inserted and connected to low intermittent suction.

Neurosurgeons were called in to evaluate A.D. They found on roentgenogram that he had a cervical dislocated fracture of C5 and C6. The thoracic and lumbar spine films revealed negative findings. The chest film revealed a lack of full lung field expansion. The blood work showed a relatively normal complete blood count and differential. The arterial gases showed signs of respiratory acidosis (pH 7.30). The chemistry panel was within normal physiological parameters. The neurosurgeons immobilized A.D.'s neck by the use of tongs (Gardner Wells). The procedure requires that two tongs be inserted into the skull above the ears at an appropriate angle to hold the neck in a position so that no further injury can occur. He was then transferred to the intensive care unit.

STUDY QUESTIONS

1. Which of the following best explains the variations in A.D.'s vital signs from those indicated in his past history?
   a. supine position
   b. spinal shock
   c. anxiety
   d. lack of mobility

2. A.D. asks you why he can feel and move his shoulders and some parts of his arms. Your response would be based on the understanding that:
   a. The concussion is causing these transient signs
   b. His injury affected the autonomic nervous center in the cerebellum
   c. These findings are consistent with the C5 and C6 level injury
   d. The brain pathways are too complex for one to know the exact etiology

3. In assessing A.D.'s respiratory status, you need to be concerned if:
   a. He does not continue taking deep breaths
   b. His anxiety causes him to have episodes of shallow breathing
   c. He is breathing only with his diaphragm
   d. His breath sounds continue to be bronchovesicular

A.D.'s respiratory status continues to improve after a battle with fluid accumulation. He is able to move 1000 ml on the incentive spirometer and is encouraged to do this every 1 to 2 hours. It has been 4 weeks since his injury. Surgery was performed 2 weeks ago and his fracture stabilized. A.D. has been unable to eat because of a severe difficulty swallowing related to the dislocation of the fractured vertebrae. He also has a paralytic ileus related to spinal shock. He has been maintained on hyperalimentation for 2 weeks and has had Dob-Hof tube feedings. He is now able to eat solid foods. He has lost about 15 pounds since admission.

4. Continued assessment of A.D.'s gastrointestinal system is important because:
   a. He may develop a stress ulcer quickly
   b. His constipation will resolve easily with the use of docusate sodium (Colace)
   c. A bowel program must begin as soon as possible
   d. Enemas will be needed every day to clear the bowel because it will not function on its own

5. A bowel program may be started because A.D.'s bowels begin to empty automatically occasionally. The most effective way to stimulate the rectum to evacuate in the quadriplegic individual is first to use:
   a. an enema at the same time every day
   b. stool softeners from admission
   c. laxatives every evening
   d. rectal suppository followed by digital stimulation

A.D. has had an indwelling Foley catheter since admission. The catheter must be checked for obstruction frequently as A.D. is unable to feel whether his bladder is getting full. A.D.'s intake of fluids must be watched carefully to prevent overloading of the vascular system. Urinary output may be low at first because of the hypotension from spinal shock.

6. Intermittent catheterization was instituted within 2 weeks after admission because:
   a. An indwelling Foley catheter will cause continued bladder infections
   b. Intermittent catheterizations will help maintain bladder tone and prevent infections
   c. Intermittent catheterization decreases stone formation
   d. An indwelling catheter interferes with the ability to gain anal sphincter control

7. A.D. is in the Rehabilitation Unit and has asked questions of a nurse about his future and his ability to have children. An accurate assessment of his sexual ability would be:
   a. He may be able to have a child but only by artificial insemination
   b. His ability to have an erection, which he now has, may indicate only that he has intact nerves to the musculature and vasculature of the penis
   c. He may indeed be able to have erections, but the necessary ejaculation may not occur for some time or may never occur
   d. This determination depends on ability of his partner to control A.D.'s spasticity

8 Cerebral Vascular Accident (CVA)

This case study will incorporate the following concepts:
1. *Etiology of cerebrovascular disease*
2. *Risk factors of cerebral vascular accident*
3. *Differentiation of types of CVA*

CASE HISTORY

Ms. R. is a 68-year-old Caucasian female.

Past History

Five years ago, she had surgery (femoral-popliteal bypass) for arteriosclerosis obliterans of her lower extremities. She has a history of smoking 1/2 to 1 pack of cigarettes a day for 50 years. She is mildly obese, weight 140 pounds, height 5 feet 2 inches. Her adult weight at age 40 was 110 pounds. She has one highball or glass of wine a day. She has been on estrogen for 20 years. Her family history is as follows: mother had adult-onset diabetes and died of cancer at age 62; father died at age 35, from an industrial accident; first sister died of subarachnoid hemorrhage, age 65; second sister, age 60, hemiparetic as the result of a CVA; two brothers died of cancer; one brother is a hypertensive diabetic; three younger sisters are alive and well.

Current Status

Ms. R. developed a severe headache 24 hours ago that was not relieved by aspirin. Several hours later, she experienced slurred speech and numbness of the fingers in her right hand, right side of her tongue, and lips. She was admitted to the neurological intensive care unit. On admission, she still had a severe right-sided headache and was very anxious.

Her vital signs were oral temperature 37° C; heart rate 90, regular beat; respirations 16, nonlabored; blood pressure, right upper extremity 230/110, left upper extremity,

225/120; pupils equal, round, reactive to light; level of consciousness on Glasgow Coma Scale of 15, speech clear; left upper extremity, normal grip; right lower extremity, weaker grip than on left; lower extremities, equal dorsiflexion; face, asymmetric smile, right facial weakness; cranial nerves, all intact; bruit over left carotid; ophthalmoscope examination, negative for papilledema and anisocoria; extraocular movements intact, no evidence of hemianopsia, negative for ptosis; ophthalmic artery pressure, decreased bilaterally. Reflexes were hyperreflexic on the right; Babinski sign, positive on the right. Lumbar puncture yielded negative result for blood, opening pressure 120; total cell count, protein, and glucose were normal. Electroencephalogram showed localized focal activity in the left hemisphere. Chest roentgenogram revealed a normal chest, no cardiomegaly. Electrocardiogram was normal. Blood studies showed clotting profiles, complete blood count, electrolytes, and triglycerides all within normal limits, except for a slightly elevated blood sugar at 140. Computed tomography (CT) scan showed increased density on the left indicating an infarction. Digital angiogram revealed a narrowing of the carotid arteries bilaterally with greater involvement on the left. Evidence of ulcerated plaques in both carotids. Middle cerebral branches indicate narrowing and occlusion on the left.

Clonidine, Prazosin hydrochloride (minipress), and hydrochlorothiazide were given to control the blood pressure. Heparin was started to maintain partial prothrombin time (PTT) at twice control levels. Additional medications prescribed were potassium chloride, docusate dosium (colace), and phenobarbital.

STUDY QUESTIONS

1. What kind of cerebrovascular accident did Ms. R. most likely experience?
   a. subarachnoid hemorrhage
   b. thrombosis with an ischemic event
   c. intracerebral hemorrhage
   d. embolic CVA

2. Ms. R.'s past history indicated some risk factors for CVA. Which of the following are risks for stroke?
   a. hypertension
   b. smoking
   c. history of family diabetes
   d. obesity
   e. estrogen therapy
   f. all of the above

3. Ms. R. was very anxious about the numbness on the right side of her mouth and tongue and the fingers of her right hand. When asked questions about these symptoms, you might appropriately respond with:
   a. Some or all of these symptoms may be temporary
   b. The part of your brain that causes these symptoms is not getting enough glucose and oxygen
   c. As soon as your blood pressure is controlled, these symptoms will disappear
   d. a, b
   e. c, d

4. After Ms. R.'s blood pressure was reduced, anticoagulation therapy was started. Current thinking about anticoagulation with heparin is that risk of further strokes is decreased because heparin interferes with the interaction of thrombin with fibrinogen and prevents conversion of prothrombin. These actions prolong whole blood clotting time. Nursing implications for heparin therapy include:
    a. checking the stool and urine for occult blood
    b. examining the individual's skin for bruises and ecchymosis
    c. checking gums and intravenous sites for bleeding
    d. reporting complaints of headache, joint pain or immobility, side or flank pain
    e. all of the above
    f. a, d only

5. A Babinski sign was present on the admission neurological examination. Which of the following statements best describes the Babinski sign?
    a. In a sitting position or lying with the thigh flexed upon the abdomen, the leg cannot be completely extended
    b. Spasmodic contracture of muscles is provoked by pressure on the nerves that led to them
    c. Flexion of the neck usually results in flexion of the hip and thigh
    d. When a moderately sharp object strokes the lateral aspect of the sole from the heel to the ball of the foot, the responses are dorsiflexion of the great toe and fanning of the small toes, indicating upper motor neuron disease

6. A bruit auscultated over the carotid artery indicates:
    a. a defective mitral valve where emboli are formed and then carried to the brain by way of the carotids
    b. unilateral complete occlusion of the carotid artery
    c. a narrowing of the carotid artery associated with atherosclerosis of the lumen
    d. a normal finding in adults after carotid endarterectomy

7. Ms. R. is discharged with medications for treating hypertension and platelet aggregation. She will return in 1 month for bilateral carotid endarterectomy surgery. What are the factors that indicate that Ms. R. should benefit from such a procedure?
    a. hypertension
    b. family history of diabetes
    c. restoration of normal perfusion pressure to the internal carotid system by surgery
    d. no known heart disease

Ms. R. recovered from her surgery. She adopted the following behaviors: stopped smoking, decreased weight to 125 pounds, walks 1 mile/day, follows a low-salt diet, and uses a diuretic to control blood pressure.

9 Bacterial Meningitis

This case study will incorporate the following concepts:
  1. Etiology and pathology of bacterial meningitis
  2. Risk factors of bacterial meningitis
  3. Alterations of consciousness
  4. Increased intracranial pressure
  5. Blood-brain barrier
  6. Osmotic diuretics

CASE HISTORY

Mr. C. is a 66-year-old Caucasian admitted to the intensive care unit with the provisional diagnosis of bacterial meningitis.

Past History

Mr. C. has had a long history of multiple medical problems and has not been well for many years. Some of his primary problems include peripheral vascular disease, coronary artery disease, chronic obstructive pulmonary disease, and hepatomegaly. Mr. C. smokes 1 to 3 packs of cigarettes a day and has a 20- to 25-year history of excessive alcohol consumption. His consumption of alcohol has increased markedly since his retirement 1 year ago.

Mr. C. was brought to the emergency room by paramedics at 1:00 p.m. He was accompanied by his wife, who reported that her husband began complaining of a severe headache the previous morning. Last evening he also noted that his neck was stiff and painful with movement, especially when he tilted his head forward. He woke up confused and disoriented on the morning of his admission. He was also restless and agitated. He had become progressively more lethargic and difficult to arouse over the morning. These latter symptoms caused his wife to call the paramedics. His wife also reported that Mr. C. had had a bad "cold" for several days. His cough had become much worse the past 2 days and he also had intermittent shaking chills.

Current Status

On admission, a check of Mr. C.'s vital signs revealed blood pressure of 150/70; heart rate, 120, regular; regular respirations of 24; rectal temperature, 102° F. Physical examination revealed his skin was warm, dry, and generally pale. Neck, groin, and axillary lymphadenopathy was present. He was normocephalic, photophobia prevented complete eye examination, and there were no signs of head injury. Breath sounds were markedly decreased in the right middle lobe and right lower lobe, bronchial breath sounds were noted in the right lower lobe, and diffuse fine and coarse crackles were present bilaterally. His cardiovascular examination revealed a normal S_1 and S_2 with faint S_4, but no murmurs. Rhythm was regular. Peripheral pulses were palpable in all extremities, but the pedal pulses were weak bilaterally. There was no edema. The abdomen was flat, soft, and not tender to palpation. Bowel sounds were present and within normal limits. The liver was palpated 3 cm below the rib cage anteriorly. His level of consciousness was assessed to be 11 on the Glascow Coma Scale. He was disoriented and would not follow commands but demonstrated localization to painful stimulus. His pupils were equal at 3 mm, round, and sluggishly reactive to light. Kernig's and Brudzinski's signs were positive, and the individual assumed an opisthotonic position when stimulated. Deep tendon reflexes were symmetrical at 1. There were no known allergies.

Laboratory findings were as follows: hematocrit 42%; hemoglobin 12 g; red blood cell count 4.2 million/mm³; white blood cell count 12,000; sodium 145 mEq/L; potassium 5 mEq/L; chloride 105 mEq/L; carbon dioxide 22 mEq/L; glucose 110 mg/dl; blood urea nitrogen 12 mg/dl. Lumbar puncture findings included cerebrospinal fluid pressure at 250 mm of water (cloudy); white blood cell count 1000 (predominantly polymorphoneucleocytes [PMNs]); red blood cell count 20 to 30; protein 100 mg/dl. Gram's stain revealed gram-positive encapsulated diplococci and a large number of white blood cells (predominantly PMNs), culture and sensitivity pending. Chest roentgenogram showed right middle lobe and right lower lobe infiltrates consistent with pneumonia, and mild cardiomegaly was also noted. Gram's stain of sputum showed gram-positive diplococci.

The provisional diagnosis of pneumococcal meningitis secondary to pneumococcal pneumonia was made. An antibiotic regimen that consisted of aqueous penicillin 2.5 million units intravenously every 4 hours and chloramphenicol 1 g intravenously every 6 hours was started. These antibiotics will continue for a minimum of 14 days, unless the culture and sensitivity demonstrate a need to change antibiotics. Spinal taps will be done in 2 days and again 2 days after the antibiotics have been stopped.

Other treatments are supportive and include (1) antipyretics and tepid baths for control of temperature and (2) close monitoring of neurological signs for indications of increased intracranial pressure. Measures to control intracranial pressure include (1) elevation of the head of the bed, (2) fluid restriction, (3) maintenance of oxygenation and ventilation, and (4) osmotic diuretics as necessary. Concurrent treatment of his pneumonia includes aerosol treatments and chest physical therapy, in addition to the abovementioned antibiotics.

STUDY QUESTIONS

1. Which of the following predisposed Mr. C. to the development of meningitis?
   a. pneumonia
   b. age
   c. chronic illness
   d. poor nutrition caused by excessive alcohol intake
   e. all of the above

2. Which of the following is suggestive of a specific central nervous system infectious process in Mr. C.?
   a. cerebrospinal fluid pressure of 250 mm of water
   b. red blood cell count 20 to 30 in cerebrospinal fluid
   c. white blood cell count of 12,000 (blood)
   d. cerebrospinal fluid glucose of 30 mg/dl

3. Which of the following is the cause of the alteration of consciousness that occurred in the early stage of Mr. C.'s infection?
   a. invasion of the brain tissue by bacteria, causing infectious encephalopathy
   b. noncommunicating hydrocephalus
   c. some disorder of the cortical neurons, whose exact etiology is unknown
   d. cerebral atrophy

4. Why are antibiotics often less effective in treating central nervous system infections than other infections?
   a. They interfere with the central nervous system's own immune defense system
   b. The blood-brain barrier limits entry of the antibiotic into the cerebrospinal fluid
   c. Antibiotics serve as an additional irritant to the central nervous system, thus producing more inflammation
   d. Bacteria causing central nervous system infections are resistant to most antibiotics

After Mr. C. was in the intensive care unit about 48 hours, his condition worsened and he became progressively less responsive. Within a short time, he was comatose and unresponsive to any kind of stimulus.

5. Which of the following is the most likely cause of the deep coma that developed 48 hours after admission?
   a. invasion of the brain tissue by bacteria causing infectious encephalopathy
   b. cerebral atrophy
   c. irreversible damage to the cortical neurons, etiology unknown
   d. hydrocephalus and cerebral edema

Mr. C. was treated with osmotic diuretics and fluid restriction, and antibiotic therapy was continued. His coma gradually lightened over the next week, and by the beginning of the second week of hospitalization, he was awake and following commands, but he was still disoriented in place and time. He continued to improve and became afebrile within 5 days after admission. After 14 days the anbitiotics were discontinued and his pneumonia had also cleared. Two days after the antibiotics were stopped a spinal tap was done. The fluid remained cloudy and contained lymphocytes, but the culture and sensitivity showed no growth after 72 hours. Prolonged cerebrospinal fluid lymphocytosis is common after most types of meningitis. Mr. C. was released from the hospital 3 days later.

6. What was the primary reason for using osmotic diuretics?
   a. to remove intracellular and extracellular fluid from the brain
   b. to remove intracellular fluid to decrease blood volume and thus decrease blood pressure
   c. to increase renal perfusion and thus maintain good renal function and urine volume
   d. to prevent syndrome of inappropriate antidiuretic hormone (SIADH) secretion and maintain good urine output

10 Hyperthyroidism: Graves Disease

This case study will incorporate the following concepts:
1. *Etiology of hyperthyroidism*
2. *Negative feedback loop*
3. *Ophthalmopathy*
4. *Goiter*
5. *Basal metabolic rate*
6. *Functions of thyroid hormones*

CASE HISTORY

Ms. R. is a 30-year-old woman who has been diagnosed as having Graves disease.

Past History

Her symptoms began 2 months ago and have been increasing in intensity since then. She has lost 25 pounds, despite an increased appetite. She has noticed that her heart seems to race and pound, even when she is at rest. She has been very irritable and has suffered from bouts of diarrhea. She states that she always feels too warm, even when others say the room is cold. The collars on her clothing feel too tight and she has begun to experience blurred vision. Though she has always had a history of regular menses, she has not had a period in 2 months.

Current Status

Ms. R. is a thin, pale, anxious woman who moves restlessly around the room. Her eyes have a bulging, staring appearance, and a mass can be seen on the anterior of her neck. Her skin is smooth, warm, and moist. She is sweating profusely, though the room temperature is 66° F. Her hair is very fine and soft. She weighs 46 kg on admission, a loss of 12 kg from her normal weight. Her vital signs are as follows: oral temperature, 99° F; heart rate, 120 at rest; respirations, 20; blood pressure, 110/50. Laboratory results are as follows: triiodothyronine (T_3), 160 mg/dl; thyroxine (T_4), 20 mg/dl; cholesterol, 10 mg/dl. She undergoes a radioactive iodine uptake test with 40% uptake in 6 hours.

STUDY QUESTIONS

1. Which of the following is the most likely cause of Ms. R.'s increased thyroid function?
   a. hyperplasia of the thyroid
   b. anterior pituitary tumor
   c. thyroid carcinoma
   d. autoimmune response

2. Which of the following best explains the physiologic mechanism(s) in Ms. R.'s oversecretion of thyroid hormones?
   a. negative feedback loop involving the anterior pituitary, thyroid, and hypothalamus
   b. activation of the thyroid gland by excessive circulating iodine
   c. positive feedback loop involving the thyroid and parathyroid glands
   d. abnormal stimulation of the thyroid gland by the adrenal glands

3. Which of the following symptoms experienced by Ms. R. may *not* resolve with treatment of her hyperthyroidism?
   a. amenorrhea
   b. weight loss
   c. exophthalmos
   d. heat intolerance

4. Ms. R.'s tight collars and neck mass suggest an enlargement of her thyroid gland, known as a goiter. In which of the following thyroid states would goiter not be found?
   a. hypothyroidism
   b. euthyroidism
   c. hyperthyroidism
   d. none of the above

5. Ms. R. is very concerned about her many symptoms, and you wish to help her understand what is happening to her body. Which of the following mechanisms account for the majority of her symptoms?
   a. increased gastrointestinal transit time, decreased basal metabolic rate
   b. increased basal metabolic rate, increased oxygen consumption, sympathetic stimulation
   c. increased aldosterone production, decreased oxygen consumption, increased TSH levels
   d. parasympathetic stimulation, decreased gastrointestinal transit time

6. Ms. R.'s team would like to treat her hyperthyroidism with oral radioactive iodine. In helping her to evaluate all of her treatment options, you want to explain the purpose of each option. Which of the following best explains the action of radioactive iodine?
   a. blocks the sympathetic responses to increased thyroid hormone
   b. destroys thyroid tissue and stops production of thyroid hormone
   c. blocks the action of thyroid hormone at target organs
   d. interrupts the release of thyroid-stimulating hormone in the anterior pituitary

11 Diabetes Mellitus (DM)

This case study will incorporate the following concepts:
 1. Etiology of type I diabetes mellitus
 2. Manifestations of type I diabetes mellitus
 3. Growth and development
 4. Metabolism
 5. Acute complications of diabetes mellitus

CASE HISTORY

S.S. is an active, thin 14-year-old. She has generally enjoyed good health, with an occasional cold or bout with the flu. She has never been hospitalized. Her family history is negative except for her maternal grandmother, who has hypothyroidism.

Past History

During late fall, Mrs. S. noticed that S.S. seemed pale and less active. S.S. stated that she felt tired and began to avoid her usual school friends and activities. She even considered resigning from the cheerleading squad. She was constantly hungry and, despite adequate food and fluid intake, lost several pounds. She complained that her clothing hung on her like bags. She also noticed that she needed to use the bathroom after almost every class in school. She could not understand where all that urine was coming from. Furthermore, she was often irritable and had difficulty concentrating on her homework.

Alarmed because of her daughter's unusual behavior, Mrs. S. took S.S. to her family physician.

Current Status

S.S. is a young white female who is 5 feet tall and presently weighs 87 pounds. She has lost 7 pounds during the past 2 weeks, despite eating five to six meals daily. Her skin is pale and dry. Her vital signs are within normal limits, although her respiration and pulse rates are higher than they were on previous physical exams. She is voiding large amounts of urine every 1 1/2 to 2 hours. She is constantly both hungry and thirsty. She is also frequently fatigued.

S.S.'s symptoms suggest type I diabetes mellitus. The physician checks a fasting glucose level and finds that it is 396 mg/dl. Urine sugar is 2% and acetone is positive. A diagnosis of type I diabetes mellitus is made.

S.S. is hospitalized to regulate her insulin requirements. She is placed on an insulin pump and is taught how to adjust the insulin infusion, depending on her body's needs. She and her family are also taught dietary management and signs and symptoms of hypoglycemia and diabetic ketoacidosis. After S.S. and her parents are able to demonstrate technical competence in insulin administration, blood glucose testing, urine testing, and menu planning, S.S. is discharged from the hospital.

STUDY QUESTIONS

1. The factor that is presently thought to have the greatest effect on the development of type I diabetes mellitus in S.S.'s case is:
   a. female sex
   b. white race
   c. grandmother's hypothyroidism
   d. increasing age

2. The most likely cause of S.S.'s polyuria and weight loss before her hospitalization was:
   a. inadequate dietary intake
   b. lack of functioning insulin
   c. non-insulin-dependent diabetes mellitus
   d. lack of functioning glucagon

3. S.S. has been taught to regulate her insulin pump according to her needs and does this very well. She will most appropriately decrease the rate of insulin injection:
   a. before meals
   b. when she has a cold
   c. before cheerleading practice
   d. while studying for school exams

4. S.S. is concerned that she will never be able to have a snack with her friends after school. She should be taught that snack food can be incorporated into her diet and that her optimal diet should be:
   a. low in both fats and carbohydrates
   b. sufficient in calories to maintain normal weight
   c. high in proteins and fats
   d. high in simple carbohydrates

5. S.S. regulates her insulin successfully for several weeks. One day at school, she notices she is having difficulty concentrating, is irritable, and has blurred vision. She notes that she has neglected to readjust her insulin pump after giving herself a bolus of insulin at breakfast. S.S.'s symptoms are most likely a result of:
   a. neurological malnutrition
   b. adrenergic reaction
   c. hypersomolar hyperglycemic nonketotic coma
   d. diabetic ketoacidosis

6. S.S. becomes ill with flu. Because she is not eating, she also discontinues her insulin for several days. She begins to feel weaker and more lethargic. She voids frequently and notes the presence of acetone in her urine. When she checks her blood glucose by finger stick, she is surprised to find that her glucose is 450 mg/dl. She tells her parents, "I can't do anything right! It's as bad as it was before" Her parents take her to the local hospital. There, a diagnosis of diabetic ketoacidosis is made. S.S. has most likely developed DKA because she:
   a. is experiencing a tremendous growth spurt
   b. has not eaten anything for several days
   c. has insufficient amounts of both insulin and stress hormones
   d. has an absolute deficiency of insulin with an increase in stress hormones

7. As S.S. matures, the earliest chronic sequela she will develop will most likely be a manifestation of:
   a. microvascular disease
   b. macrovascular disease
   c. sexual disorders
   d. other endocrine dysfunction

8. S.S. does well controlling her diabetes. She finishes high school, attends college, and finds employment. She continues to seek health care appropriately. She has a routine physical exam at the age of 26. S.S. is informed that she has a renal dysfunction. The first manifestation of renal dysfunction for S.S. is most likely:
   a. development of Kimmelstiel-Wilson nodules
   b. increased serum creatine levels
   c. proteinuria
   d. decreased blood urea nitrogen level

12 Cushing Syndrome

This case study will incorporate the following concepts:
   1. Feedback mechanisms between the anterior pituitary and the adrenal gland
   2. Effects of excess cortisol on normal metabolism
   3. Factors used to control metabolic balance

CASE HISTORY

Mrs. S. is a 44-year-old Caucasian woman who was diagnosed with Cushing disease at the age of 14. She presents to the metabolic clinic for her 3-month follow-up visit.

Past History

Mrs. S. was originally diagnosed with Cushing disease at the age of 14 as a result of a work-up for delay of onset of menses. Mrs. S. was started on hydrocortisone at that time and has since been periodically monitored. Mrs. S. is married, has two teenage daughters, and has been in relatively good health throughout her life. She did experience a period of moderate depression in her early twenties. Treatment included time off from work, stress reduction counseling, and a temporary interruption of her cortisol regime. Mrs. S. is the second oldest of seven children and is the only one in the history of the family to suffer from Cushing syndrome. Past diagnostic tests have included a dexamethasone suppression test and an intravenous pyelogram (IVP) that confirmed a pituitary basis for Mrs. S.'s disease.

Current Status

On routine examination, Mrs. S. measured 5 feet tall and weighed 132 pounds. General inspection revealed a woman who appeared about the stated age, with a thick trunk and thin extremities. She has a slight " moon face "and a definite "buffalo hump." Skin on hands appears thin, with capillaries markedly visible. She has a number of bruises that she states have been appearing spontaneously over the last 2 months. There is a scar on the lower surface of her left arm as the result of a skin tear from a lawn chair about 8 months ago. She complains of weakness in both her legs and arms, which makes reaching for an object above her head difficult. Physical parameters, including blood pressure, are within normal limits. A plasma cortisol specimen that was drawn was within normal limits, as was a blood chemistry panel that included a fasting blood glucose.

After reviewing Mrs. S.'s current physical findings, it is recommended that she decrease her hydrocortisone by 25%. She is to return in 1 month for a plasma cortisol level evaluation to determine whether this decrease is still therapeutically acceptable.

STUDY QUESTIONS

1. The cause of Mrs. S.'s current symptoms are:
   a. ectopic secretion of adrenocorticotropic hormone (ACTH)
   b. excessive levels of circulating cortisol
   c. decreased adrenal androgen levels
   d. hypofunction of the adrenal cortex

2. Early diagnostic work-up of Mrs. S included a dexamethasone suppression test. On the basis of Mrs. S.'s initial diagnosis, you would expect that the test demonstrated:
   a. a dramatic decrease in urinary free cortisol
   b. no change in urinary cortisol levels
   c. increased urine osmolarity
   d. urinary cortisol decrease with high levels of dexamethasone

3. In helping Mrs. S. understand why she bruises so easily, you tell her that the underlying cause reflects her:
   a. loss of neurological sensation
   b. increased skin pigmentation
   c. protein wasting and collagen loss
   d. decreased prothrombin levels

4. Mrs. S. is overweight and asks for some recommendations to lose weight. The most appropriate response would be:
   a. It is necessary to decrease food intake appropriately and increase the amount of exercise
   b. Weight gain is an irreversible side effect of cortisone medication
   c. Decrease in medication will resolve the current weight problem
   d. A diet restricted in sodium and complex carbohydrates is needed

5. In teaching Mrs. S. what signs and symptoms to look for as complications to her disease, you need to encourage her to:
   a. seek immediate treatment for hair loss
   b. monitor her blood pressure closely
   c. get annual flu shots and avoid infections
   d. avoid stress-provoking confrontations
   e. schedule small, frequent feedings during active periods
      1. all of the above
      2. b, d, e
      3. b, c, d
      4. a, c, e

13 Iron Deficiency Anemia

This case study will incorporate the following concepts:
1. *Erythropoiesis*
2. *Oxyhemoglobin dissociation curve*
3. *Differential diagnosis of anemias*
4. *Laboratory analysis of anemias*
5. *Clinical evaluation and treatment of iron deficiency anemia*

CASE HISTORY

Ms. I. is a healthy 29-year-old white female. She was born in the United States of Greek parents. She is currently single and enjoys a successful career as a professional tennis player.

Past History

Ms. I. has never been pregnant. Her menses occurs every 28 days, with 6 days of heavy flow and cramping. She is sexually active and has used an intrauterine device (IUD) (Lippes Loop) as her form of birth control for 5 years. She has suffered from menorrhagia and dysmenorrhea for the past 17 years and takes 15 grains of aspirin every 4 hours for the 6 days of her menstrual flow each cycle. She has a prescription for Butazolidin, which she takes on a daily basis during her peak tennis playing times (9 months/year) to prevent her knees from aching excessively. She has had this prescription for 1 year. Five months ago her physician started her on Aldomet, for a moderate hypertension resistant to salt restriction, and diuretic therapy. She takes 125 mg four times a day.

Ms. I. has noted increased shortness of breath and decreased energy during the past 4 months, exacerbated during her menses. Her cardiologist noted a tachycardia on electrocardiogram, but physical and laboratory examinations 2 months ago were otherwise unremarkable. The cardiologist suggested that her symptoms were caused by either premenstrual syndrome or stress from her profession, but assured her there was nothing physically wrong.

Current Status

Today, while playing in a tournament, Ms. I. became light-headed and syncopal and was taken by paramedics to the local medical center.

The emergency room report indicates the following: temperature 98° F; heart rate 140; respirations 28; blood pressure 100/40. Slender female, 5 feet 7 inches, 110 pounds. Resting quietly, slightly nervous, but in no acute distress. Skin is warm, pale tan; conjunctiva is pale pink; tongue is smooth, with mild cracking of the lips. Heart rate is rapid and regular with grade II/VI systolic ejection murmur heard best at the apex. Lungs are clear. Neurologic pathways are intact, despite subjective complaint of weakness.

Initial laboratory results are as follows: hemoglobin 8 g/ml; hematocrit 30%; red blood cell count 43,000; mean corpuscular volume (MCV) 70; mean corpuscular hemoglobin (MCH), 18; mean corpuscular hemoglobin content (MCHC), 27. Red blood cell smear revealed microcytosis and hypochromic cells. Electrolytes were normal.

STUDY QUESTIONS

1. On the basis of the initial work-up, what types of anemia could Ms. I. most likely have?
   a. iron deficiency
   b. anemia of chronic disease
   c. hemolytic anemia
   d. B_{12} deficiency (pernicious)
   e. α- or β-thalassemia minor

The attending physician orders further blood tests to determine the type of anemia present. The results are as follows: reticulocyte count 1%; total iron binding capacity (TIBC) 600 mg/dl; folate 480 ng/ml; B_{12} 620 pg/ml; serum bilirubin 0.5 mg/dl; serum iron 30 mg/dl; serum ferritin 8 mg/L; transferrin saturation, 10%; free erythrocyte protoporphyrin (FEP) 110 mg/dl red blood cells.

2. Which of the following tests best assists Ms. I.'s physician in differentiating between iron deficiency anemia and thalassemia?
   a. decreased serum ferritin, increased TIBC, increased FEP
   b. normal folate, B_{12}, and bilirubin
   c. decreased serum iron, normal reticulocyte count
   d. decreased transferrin saturation, normal folate

3. If an oxyhemoglobin dissociation curve were plotted for Ms. I., what would it reveal?
   a. no change, a normal curve
   b. shift to the left
   c. shift to the right

4. Which of Ms. I.'s clinical signs reflects her body's attempt to compensate for the anemia?
   a. smooth tongue and cracked lips
   b. tachycardia
   c. tachypnea
   d. heart murmur

5. What is the most likely cause of Ms. I.'s anemia?
   a. dietary iron deficiency
   b. malabsorption syndrome
   c. neoplasm
   d. blood loss

Ms. I.'s physician has discontinued her ester hydrochloride (Aldomet) and started her on propranolol hydrochloride (Inderal), 10 mg twice a day. She has also discontinued the phenylbutazone (Butazolidin) and cautioned this individual about excessive aspirin use. Mecloferamate sodium (Meclomen), 50 mg by mouth every 9 hours, has been ordered for the dysmenorrhea and for the joint pain in her knees. The IUD was removed, at Ms. I.'s request, and she was fitted for a cervical cap. Hematinic therapy was ordered.

6. Which of the following would be the preferred hematinic therapy for Ms. I.?
   a. iron dextran (Imferon) 75 mg intramuscularly four times a day
   b. iron dextran (Imferon) 50 mg intravenously in 250 ml normal saline to run over 24 hours
   c. ferrous sulfate 325 mg by mouth three times a day, given with orange juice
   d. ferrous sulfate 325 mg by mouth three times a day, given with 30 ml, antacid/anti-flatulent (Mylanta)
   e. hematinic (Theragran) 1 tablet by mouth three times a day (Theragran hematinic contains vitamins A, B complex, C, E; calcium; niacin; iron; folic acid; copper; and magnesium)
   f. Two units whole blood

7. Ms. I. is experiencing constipation, nausea, and black tarry stools. Would a timed-release/enteric coated iron preparation eliminate these symptoms?
   a. yes
   b. no

8. Ms. I. plans to continue iron therapy at home. She also wishes to alter her diet to include more iron-containing foods. Which of the following food combinations should be increased in her daily diet?
   a. cereals, yellow vegetables, eggs
   b. pork, fish, milk
   c. poultry, potatoes, tea
   d. green leafy vegetables, liver, citrus fruits

9. Ms. I. was discharged after 1 week in the hospital. She was to continue taking the oral iron, twice a day. She was to adhere to an outlined diet, curtail her tennis activities, and report to her physician in 4 weeks. Which blood tests would most accurately indicate her progress?
   a. hematocrit and MCHC
   b. reticulocyte count and hematocrit
   c. hemoglobin and MCV
   d. bone marrow aspiration

14 Acute Lymphocytic Leukemia (ALL)

This case study will incorporate the following concepts:
1. *Importance of the complete blood count (CBC) with differential and platelet count during diagnosis and treatment*
2. *Risk factors*
3. *Prognostic indicators*
4. *Phases in the life cycle of a cell as they relate to chemotherapeutic drugs*
5. *Stages and purposes of the treatment protocol*
6. *Major complications encountered during treatment*

CASE HISTORY

M.M. is a 7-year-old girl who is brought in to her physician by her mother with complaints of general fatigue, anorexia, and unexplained bruises and "rash" for the past 2 weeks.

Past History

M.M. was a full-term infant of an uncomplicated pregnancy and delivery. She has never been exposed to ionizing irradiation. All immunizations are current; she has had only one childhood disease, chickenpox, at age 5. M.M. has one brother, aged 4, who is in apparent good health. The family history is unremarkable with one exception: the fraternal grandfather died at 61 from cancer of the colon.

Current Status

M.M.'s vital signs are as follows: temperature 37° C; heart rate 92; respirations 18; blood pressure 90/60. Her height and weight are in the fifty-fifth percentile. Her skin is pale, warm, and dry with ecchymoses on the extremities and trunk. The "rash" was found to be petechiae on arms and chest. Heart rate and rhythm were normal and without murmurs; breath sounds were clear and equal bilaterally. Neither spleen nor liver was palpable, however, there were three palpable nontender lymph nodes in the submaxillary chain. The pharynx was without redness or pain, the cranial nerves were intact, and reflexes were present and equal bilaterally. The CBC with differential and platelet count results were as follows: hemoglobin 8.8 g; hematocrit 26%; red blood cell count 3.1 million/mm³; white blood cell count 13,000; neutrophils 6500; basophils 130 mm³; eosinophils 360 mm³; monocytes 1170 mm³; lymphocytes 3640; blasts 10%; platelets 50,000 mm³.

M.M. was immediately referred to a pediatric oncologist and admitted to the children's hospital for diagnosis and treatment. A bone marrow aspiration, lumbar puncture, blood work (complete blood count with differential and platelet count, and hepatic and nephrotoxic function studies), and chest roentgenograms were performed. A diagnosis of acute lymphoblastic leukemia (ALL), lacking T-cell or B-cell surface markers (null cell type), was made. The null cells were found to react positively with the common acute lymphoblastic leukemia antigen-positive (CALLA-positive). There was no evidence of mediastinal or central nervous system involvement.

STUDY QUESTIONS

1. Which physical finding is most alarming to the primary care provider?
   a. complaint of general fatigue in a 7-year-old
   b. anorexia in a 7-year-old
   c. petechiae and unexplained ecchymosis
   d. three palpable lymph nodes

2. A diagnosis of leukemia was suspected from the complete blood count results on the basis of:
   a. hemoglobin of 8.8 g
   b. total white blood cell count of 13,000
   c. platelets of 50,000 mm³
   d. 10% blasts

3. Is there anything in M.M.'s history that put her at risk for leukemia?
   a. yes, her grandfather's cancer of the colon
   b. no

4. Which of the following factors would indicate an improved prognosis for M.M.?
   a. ALL, null cell, CALLA-positive
   b. her age
   c. white blood cell count of 13,000 at diagnosis
   d. absence of hepatosplenomegaly
   e. all of the above

M.M. started chemotherapy with vincristine, prednisone, and L-asparaginase. The induction phase of therapy with these drugs lasts until remission is attained. Since chemotherapeutic agents do not cross the blood-brain barrier, intrathecal methotrexate and/or cranial irradiation is given to destroy the leukemic cells in the central nervous system. This is called the sanctuary phase.

Eight weeks after diagnosis, M.M.'s bone marrow and peripheral blood smear show no evidence of leukemic cells, therefore, remission has been attained. With remission M.M. moves into the maintenance phase, during which she receives monthly medications, complete blood counts, and periodic bone marrow aspirations and lumbar punctures.

5. The rationale for the use of multiple drug therapy as opposed to single agency chemotherapy is that:
   a. Different drugs exert their effects on cells during different phases of the life cycle of a cell
   b. No drug works on more than one phase of the cell life cycle
   c. Chemotherapeutic agents are only effective against cells during cell division (mitosis)

Three months later, during one of her clinic visits, M.M.'s complete blood count results were as follows: hemoglobin 6.8 g; hematocrit 20.4%; red blood cell count 2.1 million/mm³; white blood cell count totals 340/µl; neutrophils 200 mm³; basophils 3 mm³; eosinophils 6 mm³; monocytes 30 mm³; lymphocytes 82 mm³; platelets 20,000 mm³. The physician withholds the chemotherapy dose and transfuses M.M. with 1 unit packed red blood cells and 4 units of platelets.

6. The cause of M.M.'s pancytopenia (reduction of all cellular blood elements) is:
   a. deteriorating physical status caused by the disease process
   b. a known side effect of the chemotherapy
   c. aplastic anemia resulting from the toxic effects of the chemotherapy

7. M.M. is currently at risk for which of the three major complications of treatment?
   a. anemia, disseminated intravascular coagulation (DIC), and gram-negative septic shock
   b. aplastic anemia, DIC, and infection
   c. anemia, hemorrhage, and infection
   d. anemia, hemorrhage, and shock

15 Disseminated Intravascular Coagulation (DIC) Caused by Septicemia

This case study will incorporate the following concepts:
1. *Predisposing factors*
2. *Laboratory values as aids in diagnosis*
3. *Rationale for treatment protocol*

CASE HISTORY

M.H. is a 21-year-old Mexican-American who presented to the emergency room with a gunshot wound to the head.

Past History

Before this injury, M.H. was a healthy young man with no known medical problems. His surgical history is positive for an uncomplicated appendectomy at age 12 and a stab wound to the left upper arm at age 17 that was vascularly repaired leaving him with normal neurologic and circulatory function.

Current Status

M.H. was admitted to the emergency room with a gunshot wound to the head. Visual examination suggested that a bullet entered the left temporal portion of the head and exited near the middle of the forehead. Computed tomography (CT) scan indicated severe damage to the frontal lobe and some damage to the left temporal lobe of the brain. On admission to the emergency room, M.H. was unresponsive to verbal stimuli and demonstrated signs of shock. M.H. was intubated, started on volume replacement, and transferred to the neurological intensive care unit in serious but stable condition. As part of volume replacement therapy, he received 3 units of packed red blood cells that were correctly crossmatched. His hematocrit remained stable through the night. He continued to be comatose.

This morning the nurse notices that M.H. is oozing blood from around the intravenous site. He has heme-positive aspirate in his nasogastric tube and has areas of ecchymosis on the extremities. Morning laboratory values reveal prothrombin time (PT) 27 sec; partial prothrombin time (PTT) 63 sec; platelet count 20,000 mm³. Vital signs are within normal units: blood pressure 110/72; heart rate 95; temperature 98.8° F; respirations 24.

STUDY QUESTIONS

1. Which additional laboratory values would be *most* helpful in diagnosing DIC in M.H.?
   a. red blood cells and hematocrit
   b. fibrinogen and hematocrit
   c. fibrin split products and fibrinogen
   d. fibrin split products and red blood cells

2. M.H. developed DIC most likely as a result of:
   a. head trauma with ensuing shock
   b. blood transfusions given in the emergency room
   c. past history of vascular surgery
   d. prolonged comatose state

3. M.H.'s ~~physician~~ nurse suspected DIC, knowing that it is characterized by:
   a. massive hemorrhage
   b. microvascular thrombi and systemic bleeding
   c. microvascular thrombi and deep vein thromboses
   d. microvascular fibrinolysis and consumption of clotting factors

M.H.'s head injury is stable at this point. He remains comatose but is responsive to painful stimuli. He remains on a ventilator. All signs of shock have resolved; his circulating volume is within normal limits, as evidenced by a central venous pressure of 6, heart rate of 90, and blood pressure of 110/65. M.H. continues to show signs of bleeding.

4. Which of the following blood products would be most appropriate at this point?
   a. packed red blood cells and fresh frozen plasma
   b. whole blood and platelets
   c. cryoprecipitate and fresh frozen plasma
   d. platelets and cryoprecipitate

M.H.'s coagulation factors continue to show deterioration. His prothrombin and partial prothrombin times are more prolonged, and his platelets and fibrinogen counts are further decreased. His red blood cell count and hematocrit also are decreased. The physician orders a Heparin drip at 1500 units/hr.

5. As the nurse, you would:
   a. not hang the drip because heparin is contraindicated in someone with a bleeding disorder
   b. hang the drip with whole blood running concurrently to balance heparin's effects
   c. hang the drip because you know heparin therapy is used for life-threatening DIC
   d. not hang the drip because the dose is too high for M.H.'s weight

6. Nursing care for M.H. includes:
   a. monitoring level of consciousness and urine output
   b. avoidance of intramuscular injection
   c. observance for bleeding from every tube insertion site and body orifice
   d. checking of nasogastric aspirate and urine for presence of blood at least every 4 hours
   e. all of the above

CASE STUDY 16 Hemophilia A

This case study will incorporate the following concepts:
1. *Differentiation of several disorders of hemostasis*
2. *Genetic inheritance of hemophilia*
3. *Clinical manifestations of hemophilia*
4. *Laboratory manifestations of hemophilia*
5. *Interventions for type A hemophilia*

CASE HISTORY

J.B. is a 7-year-old male brought to the emergency room by ambulance after he was involved in an automobile-pedestrian accident. He was riding his bicycle, did not look as he emerged from a side street, and was struck by a large car traveling 40 miles an hour. J.B. was thrown from his bike and landed approximately 5 feet from the point of impact. He never lost consciousness but did sustain a deep laceration of his right thigh, which was sutured as soon as he reached the emergency room.

Past History

J.B.'s mother, who accompanied him in the ambulance, reported to the emergency room staff that her son had always been healthy. There were no abnormalities during her pregnancy with him. Labor and delivery were unremarkable, although the child seemed to bleed more than expected after he was circumcised. Other than being "clumsy" and sustaining frequent bruises, he had a history that was unremarkable. Immunizations were current and he was on no medications other than daily multivitamins. When asked about her family history, J.B.'s mother reported she was adopted and knew nothing of her natural parents or siblings. J.B. has two brothers and one sister, none of whom has any health problems or bleeding disorders.

Current Status

J.B. is a 7-year-old male; alert and oriented 3 times, in moderate distress, and bleeding moderately from the sutured laceration of his right thigh despite a pressure dressing. Temperature 97° F; heart rate 120; respirations 20; blood pressure 98/60. Head examination revealed a few minor abrasions over right temple, oozing serosanguineous fluid; pupils were equal, round, and reactive to light; conjunctivae pink and moist. Abrasion of the right lower hip, bleeding moderately. Ears, nose, and throat were unremarkable. Heart, lungs, abdomen, skeleton were unremarkable. Skin was pink and warm. There were several 4 to 5-cm ecchymoses over both forearms and legs. A 1-inch ecchymosis was observed over the left buttock in the region of the gluteal fold. A 2-cm hematoma, nonfluctuant, was located in the left popliteal region. Neurological examination produced unremarkable findings. A complete blood count with platelets and differential had a completely normal result. Chemistry panel and electrolytes yielded normal findings.

STUDY QUESTIONS

1. Initial differential diagnosis for this young boy would _not_ include:
   a. iron deficiency anemia
   b. child abuse
   c. leukemia
   d. hemophilia

J.B. is admitted to the hospital, and his attending physician orders further laboratory and roentgenogram studies. The results include the following: prothrombin and thrombin times are normal; partial prothrombin time is prolonged; factor VIII assay is 15% of normal; factor IX assay is 100% normal; platelet structure and function are completely normal; skeletal roentgenogram series shows intact bony structures without evidence of recent or remote fractures.

2. On the basis of additional data, what diagnosis is most likely?
   a. von Willebrand disease
   b. type A (classic) hemophilia
   c. Christmas disease
   d. Child abuse

3. J.B.'s mother is tested for her level of factor VIII and is found to have reduced but sufficient levels, indicating she is a carrier of hemophilia. What does this indicate about her genetic makeup?
   a. Either her father had hemophilia or her mother was a carrier of hemophilia
   b. Her sons have a 50% chance of having hemophilia
   c. Her daughters have a 50% chance of being carriers of hemophilia
   d. All of the above

4. How severe is J.B.'s hemophilia?
   a. Severe
   b. Moderately severe
   c. Mild

51

5. The attending physician wishes to augment J.B.'s factor VIII level with intravenous replacement therapy. Which of the following would *not* be appropriate?
   a. packed cells
   b. fresh frozen plasma
   c. cryoprecipitate
   d. koate

6. Despite the significant benefits of clotting factor requirements, there are complications associated with this treatment. Which of the following is *not* a potential side effect?
   a. anaphylactic or allergic reactions
   b. hemolytic anemia, post transfusion
   c. hepatitis
   d. acquired immune deficiency syndrome (AIDS) and pneumocystis carinii
   e. all of the above

7. J.B.'s follow-up care would best be handled by:
   a. a hematologist specializing in hemophilia
   b. a team of physicians of various specialties
   c. a genetic counselor
   d. a multidisciplinary team of caregivers

8. What is the most important cause of morbidity for hemophiliacs?
   a. muscle spasm and flexion deformities
   b. hemarthroses with joint destruction
   c. gastrointestinal bleeds from ulcers
   d. hematuria and chronic renal failure
   e. intracranial bleeding

9. Several years later, J.B. fails to respond as quickly to factor VIII replacement therapy as he did in the past. His physician states that he has developed an inhibitor to factor VIII. Which of the following would be appropriate alternatives to the conventional factor VIII replacement?
   a. repeated plasmapheresis
   b. replacement with factor VIII
   c. replacement with factor VIII bypassing activity (FEIBA)
   d. immunosuppression with steroids
   e. megadoses of factor VIII
   f. all of the above

10. The only drug that might be given to a person with a clotting defect is:
    a. heparin
    b. aspirin
    c. indomethacin (Indocin)
    d. phenylbutazone (Butazolidin)
    e. antiallergy medication (Chlor Trimeton)

11. You are providing instruction to J.B.'s parents. Which of the following is *incorrect*?
    a. Obesity must be prevented
    b. Snow and water skiing are not recommended
    c. Diphtheria, pertussis, tetanus (DPT) and measles, mumps, and rubella (MMR) immunizations are contraindicated
    d. Tonsillitis may be followed by pharyngeal bleeding
    e. Factor VIII levels must be elevated to 50% before surgical or dental procedures

17 Hypertension Leading to Congestive Heart Failure (CHF)

This case study will incorporate the following concepts:
1. *Hemodynamics of vessels*
2. *Alterations in myocardial contractions*
3. *Host factors*
4. *Disruption in diffusion across alveolar-capillary membrane*
5. *Pressures in the heart*
6. *Alterations in cardiac conduction and rhythm*

CASE HISTORY

Mrs. B. is a 66-year-old black woman admitted to the critical care unit with a chief complaint of shortness of breath and palpitations. The physician's preliminary diagnosis was uncontrolled hypertension complicated by atrial fibrillation and congestive heart failure.

Past History

Mrs. B.'s past health history includes pertussis, as well as the usual childhood illnesses without sequelae. Her mother died when Mrs. B. was in her early twenties. Mrs. B. was married at age 24. She describes her health as being very good until the past year, although with each of her six pregnancies the midwife told her her blood pressure was "up." Her husband died 1 year ago from a "stroke," and since his death Mrs. B. has been troubled with periods when she "couldn't get enough air."

Current Status

Mrs. B. has noticed that she is particularly short of breath when lying flat. She is able to sleep with three or four pillows but prefers to sleep in a large recliner chair. Although she enjoys walking about the neighborhood and visiting with friends, she is going out less often and coming home very tired. When Mrs. B. was visiting her daughter on a cold December day, she climbed the stairs to the second floor and began to experience chest discomfort. At first she attributed her discomfort to her usual shortness of breath with exertion. She sat down at the top of the stairs to rest and "catch her breath." After 5 minutes, she was still very short of breath and noticed that she could feel her heart "pounding with a funny rhythm" in her chest. Mrs. B.'s daughter called the urgent care clinic nearby. She received instructions to take her mother to the nearest hospital emergency room.

On arrival at the emergency room, Mrs. B. was alert and oriented to person, place, and time. Her pupils were constricted, equal, and reactive to light. Her skin was cool and dry, and her mucous membranes and nail beds were pink. Mrs. B.'s systolic blood pressure was 200. Korotkoff sounds were first heard at 198 mm Hg, then there was silence until the sounds were heard again between 140 and 100 mm Hg. Her heart rate was 110, strong and irregular; respirations were 30 and labored. The cardiac monitor displayed atrial fibrillation with rapid ventricular response and frequent premature ventricular complexes.

The emergency room team followed their established resuscitation protocol. Oxygen was administered by mask at 10 L/min. Mrs. B.'s weight was estimated to be 50 kg (110 pounds). She was given an intravenous bolus of 50 mg of lidocaine (1 mg/kg) to suppress the ventricular ectopic beats. To control her blood pressure, a nitroprusside drip was started intravenously. Five minutes later, Mrs. B.'s systolic blood pressure was 160 and diastolic pressure was 95. Her cardiac rhythm still demonstrated atrial fibrillation with a rapid ventricular response. However, no ventricular ectopic complexes were seen. A 12-lead electrocardiogram showed no evidence of acute myocardial injury. Blood was drawn to check cardiac enzyme and electrolyte levels. A lidocaine drip was started intravenously. A loading dose of digoxin was given intravenously to control the ventricular response to the atrial fibrillation. The emergency room team judged Mrs. B. stable enough to be transferred to the critical care unit.

The critical care nurse receiving Mrs. B. recorded her vital signs: blood pressure 160/90; cardiac rhythm revealed atrial fibrillation with a ventricular response of 108; occasional premature ventricular complexes were noted; respirations were 28 with oxygen by mask at 10 L/min. The nurse positioned Mrs. B. in a semi-Fowler position. The nurse continued assessing her by evaluating her neurological status. Mrs. B.'s pupils were equal at 3 mm, round, and reactive to light. She was alert, oriented, and able to follow commands. She moved all of her extremities with equal strength. While listening to Mrs. B.'s chest, the nurse noted fine rales in the posterior base of both lungs. Her S_1 and S_2 heart sounds were moderate and varied in intensity with the ventricular cycle lengths. A summation S_3, S_4 gallop was present. A soft, systolic ejection murmur was heard over the aortic valve area. Mrs. B.'s central venous pressure was estimated to be 12 cm of water pressure because her jugular veins were distended to 7 cm above her sternum. No friction rubs were heard. On palpation, Mrs. B.'s abdomen was soft and without masses or organomegaly. She complained of tenderness with deep palpation of the hepatic area. Mrs. B.'s peripheral pulses were all present and equally moderate in intensity. Her skin was cool and dry. Pitting dependent edema was noted in her lower legs. Nonpitting edema was noted around her sacral area. The nurse assisted Mrs. B. to a bedside commode, where she voided 100 ml of dark amber urine that had a specific gravity of 1.025.

Mrs. B.'s electrocardiograms did not demonstrate evolution of myocardial infarction or injury. They did show persistent atrial fibrillation with gradual slowing of the ventricular response rate.

Mrs. B.'s cardiac enzyme levels did not elevate in a pattern of myocardial infarction. Her serum glutamic oxaloacetic transaminase (SGOT) and lactic dehydrogenase (LDH) levels were elevated. The cardiologist attributed this to venous congestion in her liver. The serum electrolyte levels drawn on admission showed low serum potassium and high serum sodium. Other values were within normal limits.

Mrs. B.'s cardiac rhythm converted to sinus rhythm with a rate of 80 beats/min after she received a second dose of digoxin. She was successfully weaned from the lidocaine drip. About 15 minutes after Mrs. B. converted to sinus rhythm, she commented to the nurse that she was much less short of breath and did not feel her heart "pounding." The nurse assessed Mrs. B. carefully to be certain that no arterial emboli were released from the atria now that they were contracting again. Mrs. B. was placed on oral antihypertensive therapy and successfully weaned from the nitroprusside drip.

STUDY QUESTIONS

1. Which of the following is not likely to offer an explanation for the etiology of Mrs. B.'s essential hypertension?
   a. high potassium intake
   b. high sodium intake
   c. genetic factors
   d. sympathetic nervous system activity

2. Which of the following explains why some individuals with hypertension, such as Mrs. B., develop congestive heart failure?
   a. Preload becomes so low that efficient ventricular contraction is lost
   b. Afterload becomes so low that myocardial ischemia occurs
   c. Structural changes in the cardiac valves produce abnormal hemodynamics
   d. Afterload becomes so high that the ventricles cannot maintain adequate forward flow

3. How did atrial fibrillation contribute to Mrs. B.'s shortness of breath?
   a. Loss of synchronized atrial and ventricular contraction resulted in mild pulmonary edema
   b. Her sympathetic response to stress caused her to be more anxious
   c. The dilated atria pressed on her bronchi and esophagus
   d. They are not related

4. Why did the nurses not hear Korotkoff sounds between 198 and 140 when Mrs. B.'s blood pressure was measured by cuff on admission?
   a. There was increased systemic resistance
   b. There was decreased left ventricular afterload
   c. The cardiac output was too low
   d. Blood flow was not turbulent enough to make sounds

5. Which of the following accounts for Mrs. B.'s summation gallop?
   a. mitral stenosis
   b. impaired conduction through the atrioventricular node
   c. incomplete emptying of ventricles
   d. atrioventricular valve prolapse

6. How does sodium nitroprusside reduce blood pressure?
   a. It stimulates the α-adrenergic receptors
   b. It blocks the β-adrenergic receptors
   c. It acts directly on vascular smooth muscle
   d. It reduces myocardial contractility

18 Myocardial Infarction (MI) Caused by Coronary Artery Occlusion

This case study will incorporate the following concepts:
1. *Coagulation*
2. *Thrombosis*
3. *Tissue ischemia*
4. *Pain*
5. *Anticoagulant therapy*
6. *Cardiovascular risk factors*
7. *Pathophysiology of vessel walls*
8. *Coronary atherosclerosis*

CASE HISTORY

Mr. G. was a 49-year-old white man admitted to the critical care unit with a chief complaint of chest pain. The health care provider's preliminary diagnosis was probable acute anterior myocardial infarction.

Past History

Mr. G.'s past health history included the usual childhood illnesses without sequelae. He denies any significant medical illnesses but is currently being treated for essential hypertension. He has smoked 2 packs of cigarettes a day for 25 years. He works as an air traffic controller. In addition, his father died at the age of 51 of a heart attack.

Current Status

Mr. G. was golfing with friends when he began to experience chest discomfort. At first he attributed his discomfort to the heat. Gradually the discomfort intensified to a crushing sensation in the sternal area. Mr. G. noted that the crushing sensation spread down into his left arm and up into his lower jaw. As they left the ninth hole, Mr. G. was nauseated and rubbing his chest as an expression of pain. His golf partner was concerned that Mr. G. was having a heart attack and offered to drive him home. During the drive home Mr. G. collapsed and became unconscious.

On arrival in the emergency room Mr. G. was unconscious. His pupils were dilated and sluggishly reactive to light. He did not respond to deep pain. His skin was cool, clammy, and very pale. His facial skin was slightly gray. His blood pressure was inaudible so the nurse palpated his systolic pressure as 60. He had a weak, thready, irregular pulse of 90 and respiration of 12. The cardiac monitor displayed a sinus rhythm pattern with frequent premature ventricular complexes. The emergency room team followed their established resuscitation protocol. Oxygen was administered by mask at 10 L/min. Mr. G.'s weight was estimated to be 100 kg (220 pounds), and he was given an intravenous bolus of lidocaine to suppress the ventricular ectopic beats. To support his blood pressure, a dopamine drip was started intravenously. Five minutes later, Mr. G.'s systolic blood pressure was audible at 80 and diastolic pressure was 40. His cardiac rhythm was sinus without ventricular ectopy. A 12-lead electrocardiogram recording showed evidence of an acute injury of the anterior myocardium. Blood was drawn to check cardiac enzyme and electrolyte levels.

The critical care nurse receiving Mr. G. recorded his vital signs: blood pressure was 80/40, cardiac rhythm was sinus rhythm with occasional premature ventricular complexes at a rate of 80 beats/min, respiratory rate was 14 with oxygen by mask at 10 L/min. Mr. G.'s pupils were equal, round, and reactive to light. He responded to deep pain with purposeful movement. He moved all of his extremities with equal strength. While listening to Mr. G.'s chest, the nurse noted fine rales in the posterior bases of both lungs. His S_1 and S_2 heart sounds were moderate in intensity. An S_3 gallop was present but no murmurs or friction rubs were heard. Initial urine output was 50 ml of dark, concentrated urine with a specific gravity of 1.030. Mr. G.'s peripheral pulses were all present, equal, and faint. His skin was cool and moist and no peripheral dependent edema was noted.

Initial arterial pressures were as follows: direct arterial systolic pressure 85, diastolic pressure 40 (mean 55); right atrial pressure mean 4; right ventricular systolic pressure 26, diastolic pressure 4; pulmonary artery systolic pressure 36, diastolic pressure 20 (mean 30); and pulmonary capillary wedge pressure mean 24.

Mr. G.'s electrocardiograms demonstrated evolution of myocardial infarction in the anterior myocardium. This was deduced from the following changes in the electrocardiograms: (1) elevation of the S-T segment in leads V_{1-4} of the admission electrocardiogram, (2) inversion of the T wave in leads V_{1-4} the next morning, and (3) loss of R waves and development of QS complexes in leads V_{1-4} on the third day.

Mr. G.'s cardiac enzyme levels (creatinine phosphokinase [CPK], lactic dehydrogenase [LDH], and alanine amino transferase (serum glutamic oxaloacetic transaminase [SGOT]) were elevated in the typical pattern of myocardial infarction. The serum electrolyte levels drawn on admission were all within normal limits. Serum glucose was elevated as expected, as a result of the stress response.

Because of Mr. G.'s numerous significant risk factors and the location of the infarction, the critical care team assumed that the myocardial infarction was the result of atherosclerosis in the anterior descending branch of the left coronary artery. Mr. G. was expected to have complete bedrest for a significant period of time. The physician prescribed 500 units of heparin to be given subcutaneously every 8 hours. It was hoped that this would reduce the risk of complications caused by deep vein thrombosis and pulmonary embolus.

1. Which two of Mr. G.'s alterable risk factors for atherosclerosis are most significant?
   a. age
   b. essential hypertension
   c. smoking
   d. family history of early cardiac death
   e. male sex

2. Which of the following is the earliest pathological event leading to Mr. G.'s blocked coronary arteries?
   a. lipid deposition in the tunica intima
   b. ulceration of the tunica intima
   c. cellular proliferation in fatty streaks
   d. calcification of fibrous plaques

3. According to current knowledge, what critical event probably produced Mr. G.'s myocardial infarction?
   a. dysrhythmias in which synchronization of atrial and ventricular contraction is lost
   b. complete occlusion of a coronary artery that produces myocardial ischemia for 1 hour or more
   c. narrowing of a coronary artery lumen to less than 50% of its original size
   d. structural changes in the cardiac valves that produce abnormal hemodynamics

4. What was the primary cause of Mr. G.'s chest pain?
   a. myocardial ischemia
   b. pulmonary insufficiency
   c. high cardiac output
   d. oliguria

5. Why was Mr. G.'s arterial blood pressure low and pulmonary capillary wedge pressure high, although his right atrial, right ventricular, and pulmonary artery pressures were within normal limits?
   a. increased venous return to the left atrium
   b. decreased left ventricular afterload
   c. hypovolemia from vomiting before admission
   d. left ventricular dysfunction

6. How does heparin decrease the risk of deep vein thrombosis and pulmonary embolus?
   a. It dissolves existing clots and prevents further thrombosis by enhancing fibrinolysis
   b. It prevents further thrombosis by interfering with synthesis of vitamin K in the liver
   c. It prevents further thrombosis by interfering with conversion of prothrombin to thrombin
   d. It stabilizes already formed thrombi and prevents embolization by blocking fibrinolysis

19 Cardiomyopathy

This case study will incorporate the following concepts:
1. *Etiology and pathology of congestive cardiomyopathy*
2. *Ejection fraction as a measure of contractility*
3. *Starling's law*
4. *La Place's law*
5. *Papillary muscle dysfunction*

CASE HISTORY   Mr. B. is a 45-year-old white male, with end-stage congestive heart failure from cardiomyopathy of undetermined cause, postulated to be secondary to past history of alcohol abuse. He reports decreased exercise tolerance over the last week without signs of acute congestive failure, that is, no increase in pedal edema or dyspnea on exertion; no change in sputum, which is chronically blood tinged; and no pleuritic chest pain or shortness of breath.

Mr. B. was seen in the admitting office 2 days before his admission, when a slight increase in the right lower lobe infiltrate was noted. Three years ago he had cardiac catheterization done that demonstrated an ejection fraction of between 12% and 18% with clean coronary arteries. He also has a history of chest pain that appears to be gastrointestinal in origin and a history of ventricular dysrhythmias, premature ventricular contractions (PVCs), and runs of ventricular tachycardia. Medications were started to control his dysrhythmias, but when they increased his congestive heart failure, they were discontinued. Current medications include digoxin, furosemide (Lasix), spironolactone (Aldactone), crystalline warfarin sodium (Coumadin), diazepam (Valium), and isosorbide dinitrate (Isordil).

Past History

Cardiomyopathy with biventricular failure of 6 years' duration and history of alcoholism. No surgical history to date. Mr. B.'s mother has cancer and his father died of congestive heart failure and chronic obstructive pulmonary disease (COPD). There is no family history of diabetes, hypertension, tuberculosis, or renal disease. Mr. B. retired 6 years ago and lives with his wife. He denies alcohol ingestion for the last 5 years but has smoked 1 1/2 packs of cigarettes a day over a period of 30 years.

Current Status

Mr. B. is a generally cachectic white male in no acute distress at this time. His blood pressure is 90/76, heart rate 100, temperature 98° F. His weight is 110 pounds. Positive findings on physical examination include the following: chest expansion is symmetrical with inspiration, and bibasilar crackles without wheezes are present; jugular venous pressure is about 8 cm water; cardiac auscultation reveals S_1 and S_2 with a summation gallop and a grade II/VI holosystolic murmur at the left sternal border, apex, and axilla. His pulses are 2+/4, all present, and there is trace to 1+ edema in both feet. The liver is percussed 8 to 10 cm below the costal margin.

Laboratory findings reveal the following: hemoglobin 14.4 g; hematocrit 44.4%; white blood cell count 11.2 k/mm³; prothrombin time 38 (11 control); partial prothrombin time 103 (32 control); sodium 124 mEq/L; potassium 3.6 mEq/L; chloride 88 mEq/L; carbon monoxide 24 (normal in smokers is 4% to 5% of total hemoglobin); blood urea nitrogen 24 mg/dl; creatinine 1.2 mg/dl; glucose 214 g/dl. Arterial blood gases on room air are Po_2 62 mm Hg, Pco_2 29 mm Hg, pH 7.49, bicarbonate 21 mEq/L.

Electrocardiogram showed normal sinus rhythm, rate 100/min, axis of -70 left axis deviation, PR interval 0.21, QRS 0.16, left bundle branch block (LBBB) with left ventricular hypertrophy and left atrial enlargement. Chest roentgenogram shows a slight increase in a chronically present right lower lobe infiltrate with slight increase in bilateral pleural effusions since the last chest roentgenogram.

STUDY QUESTIONS

1. Normal ejection fraction is 50% to 70%; Mr. B.'s ejection fraction is 12% to 18%. Which of the following most likely accounts for this decrease?
   a. decreased ventricular compliance
   b. ventricular dysrhythmias
   c. decreased contractility
   d. increased heart rate

2. Which of the following factors is important in determining Mr. B.'s cardic output?
   a. ventricular dilatation
   b. blood volume
   c. heart rate
   d. all of the above

3. Mr. B. was on crystalline warfarin (coumadin) therapy to:
   a. prevent thrombophlebitis in the lower extremities resulting from sluggish blood flow
   b. prevent narrowing of the coronary arteries caused by plaque formation and sluggish circulation
   c. prevent thrombus formation within the chambers of the dilated heart
   d. make blood less viscous and, therefore, reduce the work load on the heart

4. Mr. B. has a holosystolic murmur because:
   a. the valvular regurgitation is caused by papillary muscle dysfunction
   b. the valve leaflets become heavily laden with calcium deposits and become stenotic
   c. the heart valve leaflets enlarge with the disease process and cause the valves to become incompetent
   d. ventricular dysrhythmias create turbulent blood flow around the aortic root

5. The primary cause of Mr. B.'s ventricular dysrhythmias was:
   a. low serum potassium secondary to the diuretic therapy
   b. myocardial muscle disease
   c. myocardial muscle irritability secondary to digoxin use
   d. myocardial irritability secondary to stress and anxiety

20 Hypovolemic Shock

This case study will incorporate the following concepts:
1. *Etiology of hypovolemic shock*
2. *Compensatory mechanisms*
3. *Signs and symptoms of shock*
4. *Hemodynamics of shock*

CASE HISTORY

Mr. C. is a healthy 20-year-old male who was injured in an industrial accident, causing him to suffer a crushed pelvis, ruptured spleen, and associated blood loss.

Past History

Mr. C. has an unremarkable history other than childhood diseases. He has not suffered any previous traumatic injuries and has no chronic illnesses. He has been in good health, exercises daily, is 6 feet tall, and weighs 165 pounds.

Current Status

At midnight Mr. C. was working at an oil rig when a 10-ton forklift fell off its blocks onto him, pinning him at the pelvis. He was trapped for approximately 20 minutes while a crane was secured to remove the forklift. Paramedics at the scene started intravenous lactated Ringer's solution at 150 ml/hr. Vital signs were also obtained: heart rate 120; blood pressure 90/70; respirations 46. His level of consciousness was reported as awake and complaining of pelvic, back, and abdominal pain. He was pinned face down and has reduced movement of his lower extremities. His toes were mottled, pedal pulses were absent, radial pulses weak, brachial and carotid pulses palpable.

Mr. C. had a supraventricular tachycardia by electrocardiogram monitor and reported that his heart was "pounding in his chest." He was tachypneic and became short of breath with conversation. He was restless and continued to complain of pain. He was pale but did not show any cyanosis. Peripheral pulses were absent with the exception of a thready brachial pulse; a Doppler was required for blood pressure; skin was cool and clammy; petechiae were present over his upper thorax, face, and neck.

On transport to the hospital the vital signs noted were as follows: heart rate 138, blood pressure 88/70, respirations 46, and confusion. He was diagnosed as being in hypovolemic shock (extracellular fluid volume deficit), and his intravenous fluids were increased to 300 ml/hr while blood samples were sent for type and cross-match, and chemical and hematologic analysis.

Roentgenograms revealed lobar collapse, normal cervical spine (C-spine) (visualized to C-7), and displaced unstable pelvic fracture (iliac crest, sacroiliac joint, and pubic rami). Initial hemoglobin was 9 g and hematocrit was 30 ml. Blood gas results were as follows: Po_2 41 mm Hg; PCO_2 47 mm Hg; pH 7.38, oxygen saturation 71% on room air. Oxygen was started at 3 L/min by nasal cannula and repeat blood gases were Po_2 84 mm Hg, PCO_2 35 mm Hg, pH 7.45, and oxygen saturation 96%.

An indwelling Foley catheter was inserted with return of 200 ml of amber colored urine. Urine output measured over the next hour was 40 ml. Abdominal lavage revealed peritoneal fluid with significant red blood cells.

Mr. C.'s condition improved after resuscitation of 1000 ml lactated Ringer's and 2 units of red blood cells over 1 hour; heart rate 110, blood pressure 102/70, respirations 28. Chemistry results included the following: sodium 137 mEq/L, chloride 110 mEq/L, potassium 3.6 mEq/L, creatinine 1.0 mg/dl, glucose 276 mg/dl whole blood, and amylase 36 somogyi units/dl.

He was then taken to the operating room for surgical correction of a ruptured spleen; there he received 6 additional units of blood and was admitted to the intensive care unit with the following vital signs: heart rate 104, blood pressure 106/70, respirations 26. He was extubated and placed on 40% oxygen by face mask. He was in pelvic traction to stabilize his fractures. His continuing additional active medical problems included retroperitoneal hematoma not drained in the operating room, increased temperature, bibasilar atelectasis, and decreased urine output.

STUDY QUESTIONS

1. Mr. C.'s extracellular fluid volume deficit occured as a result of which primary mechanism?
   a. decreased intake of fluids and electrolytes
   b. excessive loss of blood and fluids
   c. shifts of fluids and electrolytes into nonaccessible areas

2. Which of Mr. C.'s signs are the result of compensatory mechanisms directed at maintaining cardiac output?
   a. increased heart rate and oliguria
   b. decreased blood pressure and sodium loss
   c. respiratory acidosis and decreased heart rate
   d. all of the above

3. The mechanism *most* responsible for Mr. C.'s tachycardia is:
   a. hypoxemia caused by atelectasis
   b. anxiety as a result of traumatic injuries and pain
   c. secretion of epinephrine and norepinephrine in response to decreased blood pressure
   d. reaction to blood transfusion

4. What is the best explanation of Mr. C.'s initial blood gas results?
   a. respiratory alkalosis
   b. decreased tissue perfusion
   c. compromised lung capacity
   d. increased alveolar perfusion

5. Mr. C.'s high glucose level is the result of:
   a. rapid infusion of lactated Ringer's solution
   b. infusion of 2 units of red blood cells
   c. decreased urinary output
   d. compensatory mechanism in response to stress

21 Ventricular Septal Defect (VSD)

This case study will incorporate the following concepts:
1. *Hemodynamics*
2. *Etiology of ventricular septal defect*
3. *Risk factors of ventricular septal defect*
4. *Congestive heart failure in infancy*
5. *Cyanosis*
6. *Heart sounds and murmurs*

CASE HISTORY

A.B. is a 3-month-old boy who was born with a ventricular septal defect (VSD).

Past History

A.B. was the product of a full-term pregnancy. He is the first child of a 43-year-old mother and a 45-year-old father. His family history is negative except that both paternal grandparents have essential hypertension, and his materal grandfather has arteriosclerotic heart disease. He also has a male paternal cousin who died at 2 months of age with trisomy 18 and VSD.

At 2 weeks of age, a heart murmur that indicated VSD was heard. A.B. was acyanotic at that time and had gained a few ounces over his birth weight. Subsequently he failed to gain weight adequately, and his parents had an increasingly difficult time feeding him. It was difficult for him to suck and to swallow his formula. He became very tired during feedings and took 45 minutes to an hour to consume 1 ounce of formula. He seemed to get very short of breath while eating and was irritable when awake. He was admitted to the hospital for further diagnosis and treatment.

Current History

A.B. is a small baby. He has gained only half the weight expected for his age. He has a weak cry, which is frequently interrupted by his gasping for air. He is irritable and hard to comfort. His skin feels damp, even when he is dressed only in a diaper. He is generally pale with circumoral cyanosis. Heart rate is 180, respirations 60. He has hepatomegaly; the liver was palpated at 4 cm below the costal margin. A.B. has a precordial bulge and a grade III/VI systolic murmur heard along the left lower sternal border with a systolic thrill.

An electrocardiogram reveals biventricular enlargement; chest roentgenogram shows cardiac enlargement with increased pulmonary arterial markings; cardiac catherization and angiogram show a large (3 cm) VSD visualized in the membranous and muscular septum. Intraventricular pressures are equal at systemic levels. Computed resistances show that systemic vascular resistance is greater than pulmonary vascular resistance. Oximetry shows that oxygen saturation is greater in the right ventricle than in the right atrium, greater in the left ventricle than in the right ventricle, and equal in the left ventricle and left atrium.

STUDY QUESTIONS

1. Which of the following most likely accounts for A.B.'s cyanosis?
   a. shunting of the blood through his VSD
   b. congestive heart failure
   c. failure to thrive
   d. his dyspnea

2. Which of the following risk factors is probably most closely linked to the development of A.B.'s VSD?
   a. grandparents' hypertension
   b. cousin's trisomy 18
   c. mother's age
   d. father's age

3. In a large VSD, such as A.B.'s, which of the following determines the direction of the blood flow through the shunt?
   a. size of the VSD
   b. pressure difference between the ventricles
   c. location of the VSD
   d. relative difference between pulmonary and systemic resistance

4. Why was A.B.'s heart murmur not detected immediately after he was born?
   a. VSD was not present at birth
   b. Heart size was too small to transmit sound
   c. Murmur was too low-pitched to be heard
   d. Pulmonary and systemic resistance were equal

A.B. is treated for congestive heart failure with digoxin and diuretics. He returns home on this regimen and slowly gains weight. His color has improved and he is no longer cyanotic. He still tires easily during feedings but is less tachypneic or tachycardic now. Nonetheless controlling his congestive heart failure is difficult and surgery is delayed. Repeated cardiac catheterizations show that A.B. is experiencing gradually increasing pulmonary hypertension, manifesting as increased pulmonary vascular resistance. When

A.B. is 3 years old, he is readmitted to the hospital for a cardiac catheterization and closure of his VSD.

A.B. is again cyanotic on admission. He is dyspneic on exertion, such as active playing, but is not dyspneic at rest. He is still small for his age, but his development is normal. Blood pressure is 100/60, heart rate 110, respirations 24.

His electrocardiogram shows cardiomegaly and biventricular enlargement; chest roentgenogram shows an enlarged heart; cardiac catheterization and angiogram reveal a 3-cm VSD with oxygen saturation greater in the left atrium than in the left ventricle and pressures in the ventricles equal. Pulmonary vascular resistance is greater than systemic vascular resistance.

5. Which of the following factors most likely accounts for A.B.'s cyanosis now?
   a. poorly controlled congestive heart failure
   b. direction of blood flow through VSD
   c. poor nutritional status
   d. VSD increased in size

22 Emphysema

This case study will incorporate the following concepts:
 1. Muscles used in ventilation
 2. Elastic recoil of chest wall
 3. Airway resistance
 4. Arterial blood gases
 5. Tidal volume
 6. Oxyhemoglobin dissociation curve

CASE HISTORY

Mr. T. is a 65-year-old man who is the vice president of a prestigious law firm. As a result of the stressful nature of his job, Mr. T. has a habit of smoking 2 packs of cigarettes a day and has done so for the past 35 years.

Past History

During the last few years Mr. T. has experienced slight shortness of breath and a mild cough with activity and on arising in the morning. Recently, Mr. T. has noticed that he has difficulty climbing the stairs at work, which not only produces fatigue but often requires him to stop at varying intervals so that he may catch his breath. He has also noticed that besides being short of breath with exertion, he tends to experience dyspnea at rest. He has had an approximate weight loss of 10 pounds within the last 2 months. Mr. T. is brought into the emergency room by his wife for evaluation because of his increasing dyspnea and because he must sleep sitting up with the aid of several pillows.

Current Status

On admission to the emergency room, Mr. T. is a thin, frail-looking man in acute respiratory distress. He is restless and tachypneic and uses pursed lip breathing. He is sitting on the side of the bed, leaning on an over-the-bed table. His vital signs are as follows: heart rate 120, respirations 30, blood pressure 140/80. A chest roentgenogram is taken and arterial blood gases are drawn on room air. Mr. T.'s arterial blood gases indicate the following: PO_2 39 mm Hg; PCO_2 52 mm Hg; pH 7.32, bicarbonate 36 mEq/L. He is now placed on 2 L of nasal oxygen and is sent to the medical intensive care unit for further evaluation and treatment.

The chest roentgenogram reveals a flat, low diaphragm and hyperinflation of the lungs. The lung fields are relatively clear but appear translucent, and no gross cardiac enlargement is seen. Auscultation of the lungs reveals decreased breath sounds with expiratory wheezes. Mr. T.'s chest has an increased anteroposterior diameter, and the accessory muscles are used for ventilation. Pulmonary function tests reveal decreased tidal volume, decreased vital capacity, increased total lung capacity, and prolonged forced expiratory volume. Arterial blood gases are redrawn on 2 L of oxygen. The results are as follows: PO_2 49 mm Hg, PCO_2 50 mm Hg, pH 7.25, bicarbonate 32 mEq/L.

It is felt that Mr. T. could benefit from a respiratory treatment so a nebulizer treatment with bronchodilators is given to him. After the treatment Mr. T.'s lungs are reauscultated, and it is noted that his wheezes are decreased, he is now less restless, and his respiratory rate has decreased to 22. Arterial blood gases are now redrawn after the treatment and the results now reveal PO_2 of 58 mm Hg, PCO_2 42 mm Hg, and pH 7.38.

After a few days in the intensive care unit, Mr. T. is transferred to a medical floor, where he receives rigorous pulmonary toilet, counseling on how to stop smoking, and breathing retraining through the use of effective pursed lip breathing. After 1 week it is felt that Mr. T. can return home with the use of home oxygen at 2 L/min. A visiting nurse will follow him at home for periodic checkups and consultation.

STUDY QUESTIONS

1. Which of the following is the most likely cause of Mr. T.'s dyspnea?
   a. increased lung compliance
   b. decreased elastic recoil
   c. decreased lung compliance
   d. increased elastic recoil
   e. a, b
   f. a, d
   g. b, c
   h. c, d

2. The causes of Mr. T.'s barrel chest would include:
   a. excessive secretions
   b. severe hypoxemia
   c. hyperinflation of the lungs
   d. thickening of bronchial mucosa

3. Retention of carbon dioxide in individuals with chronic obstructive pulmonary disease (COPD), such as Mr. T., is caused by what mechanism?
   a. hyperventilation
   b. dilatation of the bronchial tree
   c. hypoventilation
   d. hypoxemia

4. Oxygen given to individuals with COPD should be administered in the following way:
   a. high concentration
   b. low concentration
   c. varying pH levels
   d. varying carbon dioxide levels

5. Which of the following best explains Mr. T.'s weight loss?
   a. Cigarette smoking decreases his sense of taste, thus decreasing his appetite
   b. COPD increases the body's need for calories
   c. Cigarette smoking increases the basal metabolism rate, leading to weight loss
   d. COPD prevents the body from using nutrients

23 Bronchopneumonia in the Elderly

This case study will incorporate the following concepts:
1. *Differential diagnosis*
2. *Diagnosis of pneumonia in the elderly*
3. *Treatment of pneumonia*
4. *Complications*
5. *Prevention*

CASE HISTORY

Mr. B. is an 88-year-old white male. He owns his own home and has a 50-year-old care-giver who lives in the home. Currently Mr. B. walks with a walker and takes daily strolls around the block with the caregiver. He is able to perform all activities of daily living, with the exception of preparing meals, which the caregiver does. Medications include a diuretic for hypertension and a stool softener.

Past History

Mr. B. has mild left hemiparesis caused by a stroke 5 years ago. He has had an upper respiratory infection for the past 3 weeks. Over the past 3 days Mr. B. has become pro-gressively weaker and more lethargic. Last night he was unable to complete his walk around the block. The caregiver reports that he had one episode of falling while going to the bathroom last week and was also incontinent and confused last night. Although Mr. B. has voiced no specific complaints, the caregiver has become concerned by his reduc-tion in daily activities and inability to get rid of his "cold." The caregiver has brought him into the clinic for evaluation.

Current Status

Mr. B. appears to be his stated age. He is well groomed and neat, uses a walker for ambulation, and walks with a noticeable limp. He answers all questions asked of him appropriately but with much effort. Mucous membranes are moist. Blood pressure is 142/80, heart rate 100, respirations 24, temperature 98.4° F.

The electrocardiogram shows normal sinus rhythm. Chest roentgenogram shows previous scarring and small infiltrates in the right lower lobe and left lower lobe. Skin is warm and dry. Eyes are watery. Nose and throat have inflamed, irritated mucous membranes. Thorax and lungs show diaphragmatic excursion adequate for stated age, breath sounds bronchial, and percussion is normal and resonant. Cardiac examination shows point of maximal impulse (PMI) at the fifth intercostal space; S_1, S_2, and S_4 are heard. Mental status is lethargic and cooperative. The laboratory report is within normal limits: blood sugar is 140 mg; urinalysis shows no bacteria or pyuria.

STUDY QUESTIONS

1. Which of the following most likely accounts for Mr. B.'s lethargy?
   a. hypertension
   b. infection
   c. diabetes
   d. digitalis toxicity

2. Which of the following complicates the diagnosis of pneumonia in Mr. B.?
   a. His stroke has caused a decrease in lung function
   b. Fever, tachycardia, and increased respirations are often not present
   c. The microorganisms causing pneumonia in the elderly create atypical symptoms
   d. The elderly have increased sputum production that masks the symptoms

Mr. B. has shown little improvement over the last 24 hours and is now having some dyspnea and coughing up of rust-colored sputum. Sputum and blood cultures have been sent to diagnose the microorganism causing his illness and to help identify the proper treatment regimen. A complete blood count was repeated, showing a white blood cell count of 18,000. Hydration was increased, and a repeated chest roentgenogram now indicates definite right lower lobe and left lower lobe filtrates. Breath sounds are bronchial. Percussion now is dull over the right lower lobe and left lower lobe. Pencillin (Penicillin G Potassium) is started until the sputum cultures return.

3. In addition to appropriate antibiotic therapy, other measures are necessary in the elderly to prevent pulmonary complications of necrosis, lung abscess, and empyema. Which other therapeutic measure(s) might be necessary for Mr. B.?
   a. hydration and chest physiotherapy
   b. bedrest
   c. nebulizers
   d. cough suppressants and expectorants

4. Mr. B.'s rust-colored sputum is indicative of:
   a. hemorrhage in his lung tissue
   b. *Streptococcus pneumoniae* in his lungs
   c. stasis of pulmonary secretions
   d. deposition of fibrin on the pleural surfaces

Mr. B. is continued on penicillin (Penicillin G Potassium) every 6 hours after his sputum culture confirms that the microorganism causing his pneumonia is *S. pneumoniae*.

5. Blood cultures were drawn because Mr. B. was at risk for the development of sepsis (bacteria in the blood stream). Which of the following factors helps to explain his increased risk?
   a. slower immune response
   b. decreased mucociliary function
   c. delayed diagnosis of infection
   d. all of the above

Mr. B.'s condition is improving. He is continuing on penicillin (Penicillin G Potassium) every 6 hours, fluids, and pulmonary physiotherapy. He is able to resume his normal level of activity. After 10 days of antibiotic therapy, his breath sounds are vesicular and the chest roentgenogram result is negative.

6. What would you recommend for Mr. B. to prevent pneumonia in the future?
   a. Have an influenza immunization
   b. Have annual influenza and pneumococcal immunizations
   c. Obtain a pneumococcal immunization
   d. Have influenza immunization every year and pneumococcal immunization every 5 years

24 Cystic Fibrosis (CF)

This case study will incorporate the following concepts:
1. Exocrine system
2. Etiology of cystic fibrosis
3. Respiratory impact of cystic fibrosis
4. Malnutrition
5. Heart failure, pulmonary hypertension

CASE HISTORY

S.S. is a 7-year-old Caucasian girl who was diagnosed as having cystic fibrosis (CF) when she was 3 months old.

Past History

S.S. is the second child born to a 33-year-old father and a 28-year-old mother. Her sister is a well child. A maternal uncle died in his midteens of pneumonia secondary to cystic fibrosis. The rest of the family history is negative (see the figure below).

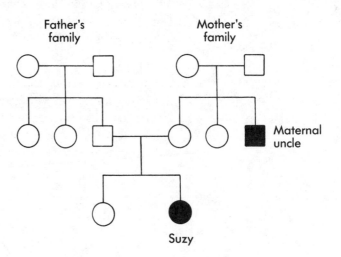

S.S. has consistently had a poor appetite and difficulty maintaining adequate weight gain. This is her tenth hospitalization for pneumonia in the past 12 months. She has recently started complaining of headaches, which are relieved by oxygen through nasal cannula at a flow rate of 2 L. S.S. has complained of increased congestion, increased sputum production, and decreased tolerance for exercise.

Current Status

S.S. has thick, tenacious respiratory secretions. She has no hemoptysis. Stools are fatty and foul-smelling and she normally stools twice a day. She weighs 15.9 kg and she is 3 feet 10 1/2 inches tall. She tries to eat high-calorie foods but is not interested in food or eating. She is a pretty, petite blond child. She is noticeably thin, has a quick grin, and has pale skin. S.S. displays familiarity with the hospital unit and roams it quite freely.

Positive findings of physical examination include the following: crackling breath sounds on inspiration, poor appetite, smallness for age and height, and moderate clubbing in fingers. There is no cyanosis, though pallor is noticeable; there is no edema, hemoptysis, or diarrhea; and the abdomen is soft to palpation. S.S. has a Hickman catheter in place.

The diagnosis is cystic fibrosis, with Pseudomonas pneumonia and poor nutrition. Chest roentgenogram demonstrates chronic lung disease and early emphysema. Ear oximetry saturations were above 90% with oxygen flow rate at 2 L. Chest physiotherapy 5 times/day. Medications include pancrelipase (Cotazym-S), (Vi-Daylin F), vitamin E, terbutaline sulfate, tobramycin sulfate, and heparin flush after each dose of intravenous medication. Tobramycin sulfate levels were within the therapeutic range and electrolytes were within normal limits.

STUDY QUESTIONS

1. Which of the following best explains why S.S. has cystic fibrosis?
   a. failure to thrive
   b. age of parents at time of S.S.'s birth
   c. family genetic pedigree
   d. result of frequent infections

2. Why would you expect S.S. to be poorly nourished?
   a. malabsorption of fats and proteins
   b. deficiency of fat-soluble vitamins
   c. high calorie expense of breathing
   d. all of the above

3. Why is S.S. receiving antibiotics?
   a. prophylactically to prevent respiratory infections
   b. to break the infectious process
   c. to prevent infection of the Hickman catheter
   d. to decrease the normal flora in her airways

4. S.S. receives chest physiotherapy to:
    a. facilitate air exchange
    b. strengthen chest muscles
    c. loosen secretions from lungs and move them out of the airways
    d. a, c
    e. b, c

5. Which of the following would you expect as S.S.'s disease progresses?
    a. respiratory infections, dyspnea
    b. failure to thrive, meconium ileus equivalent
    c. development of a barrel chest
    d. all of the above

6. Pulmonary hypertension and right ventricular hypertrophy are seen with this disease. What symptoms might S.S. demonstrate that would indicate these complications?
    a. increased respiratory distress
    b. tachycardia
    c. edema
    d. increased coughing
    e. a, c, d
    f. a, b, c

25 Asthma

Thi case study will incorporate the following concepts:
  1. *Bronchial tone and bronchoconstrictor forces*
  2. *Sites of drug action and bronchodilating forces*
  3. *Pathological changes of asthma*
  4. *β-Adrenergic hyporesponsiveness*
  5. *β-Adrenergic blockade*
  6. *IgE sensitization*
  7. *Degranulization of mast cells*
  8. *Pharmacological management of asthma*
  9. *Immunogenetics*
  10. *Smooth muscle receptors: α- and β-cholinergic*

CASE HISTORY

Past History

D.K., age 3, was a product of a normal pregnancy and delivery. His birth weight was 6 pounds 7 ounces. Throughout most of infancy and at present, D.K. has been around the tenth percentile for weight and the twenty-fifth percentile for height. He has no known allergies at present but was taken off formula and placed on (Prosobee) because of eczema. His mother and father both have pollen allergies, and his brother, age 9, has asthma. He is currently on no medications and no special diet. His brother had an upper respiratory infection 2 weeks ago and was hospitalized for an acute asthma episode.

Current Status

D.K. was admitted to the hospital emergency room at 3:00 a.m. in acute respiratory distress. Two hours before admission, D.K. had awakened with a tight nonproductive cough, low-grade fever, and shortness of breath. His mother tried to alleviate the symptoms with steam and fluids but he continued having difficulty breathing. He was pale, was unable to cry, and could only speak in short, panty phrases so she rushed him to the hospital. Examination revealed malar fushing, intercostal and substernal retractions, audible expiratory wheezing, and nasal flaring. Chest examination revealed prolonged expiratory phase throughout his chest and hyperresonance over the lung fields. Vital signs on admission were as follows: temperature 37.8° C; respirations 48, labored and irregular; heart rate 138; blood pressure 104/60; weight 11.7 kg. Diagnosis was acute asthma episode and rule out bronchiolitis.

D.K. was given 0.2 ml of epinephrine 1:1000 subcutaneously twice with no response. Terbutaline sulfate treatment 1 ml in 2.5-ml normal saline by nebulizer was given with little response. An intravenous drip was started with D_5W in 0.45 normal saline at 30 ml/hr. To enhance the therapy, the following medications were given: an immediate intravenous loading dose of aminophylline, followed by a continuous intravenous maintenance dose; intravenous hydrocortisone sodium succinate for injection (Solu-Cortef) was also ordered. Laboratory values were normal except the following: white blood cells 20,000, eosinophils 7%, basophils 2%. Arterial blood gases on room air were the following: pH 7.34, PCO_2 46 mm Hg; carbon dioxide 30 mEq/L. Chest roentgenogram showed no atelectasis. Other orders included use of cold air humidifier, chest physiotherapy every 4 hours, 2 L oxygen by nasal cannula, high Fowler position, and clear, room-temperature fluids. By the second day of hospitalization, D.K. was advanced to a soft diet and changed to aminophylline and albuterol by mouth. By the third day he was breathing much more easily and discharged with a prescription for anhydrous theophylline (Theo-dur) and metaproterenol sulfate (Alupent) syrup.

STUDY QUESTIONS

1. What factor in D.K.'s history is most strongly associated with his developing asthma?
   a. delayed growth pattern
   b. history of infantile eczema
   c. positive familial history
   d. allergic history to milk products

2. The immunoglobulin (Ig) most active in the underlying pathophysiology of asthma is:
   a. IgM
   b. IgG
   c. IgE
   d. IgA

3. Which of D.K.'s symptoms are commonly experienced in an acute asthma attack?
   a. dyspnea and wheezing
   b. lethargy and decreased inspiratory phase
   c. hypotension and nonproductive cough
   d. fever, rales, and hypoventilation

4. Which clinical sign would indicate ventilatory failure in D.K.?
   a. paroxysmal sneezing
   b. decrease in wheezes
   c. diaphoresis
   d. nonproductive cough

5. Aminophylline was given to D.K. to:
   a. decrease inflammation
   b. dilate the bronchioles
   c. enhance the antigen-antibody reaction
   d. prevent infection

6. D.K.'s white blood cell count is elevated, suggesting that the impetus for his attack was related to:
   a. excessive physical therapy
   b. contact with an allergen
   c. viral or bacterial infection
   d. immune incompetency

26 Urolithiasis

This case study will incorporate the following concepts:
1. *Risk factors for developing urolithiasis*
2. *Clinical and laboratory manifestations associated with urolithiasis*
3. *Conservative and surgical interventions*
4. *Nutrition and prevention of renal calculi*

CASE HISTORY

Mr. G. is a 42-year-old farmer from Texas. For the past week he has noted "twinges" in his right lower back. At 3:00 a.m. today, he awoke with excruciating pain in his back, unresponsive to a hot water bottle, bag balm liniment rub, or aspirin. He spent 4 hours pacing the house with intermittent bouts of emesis. Finally his wife persuaded him to go to the emergency room 2 hours away.

Past History

While pacing in the emergency room examining room, Mr. G. reported good health in the past with no prior medical illnesses or surgical procedures. He takes no medications, does not use tobacco or alcohol, and is very active on the farm, working 12 to 14 hours a day. He denied any recent or remote trauma.

Family history revealed that the individual was raised in a rural Texas hamlet. His family was healthy, although his father and grandfather occasionally "passed blood in their water." No cause for this problem was ever sought.

Current Status

Physical examination revealed a healthy-appearing Caucasian male, appearing somewhat older than stated age, pacing and wincing in acute discomfort. Vital signs were as follows: temperature 97° F; heart rate 140, respirations 28, blood pressure 138/78.

Findings included cool and moist skin, moderate to severe right flank, and abdominal pain without rebound tenderness. Mr. G. vomited three times during the examination. His complete blood count revealed a modest elevation in white cells (10,800) with 3% bands, 29% lymphocytes, 1% eosinophils, 1% basophils, 6% monophils, 60% segmented neutrophils, 0 band cells. Hemoglobin was 14.8 g, hematocrit 42%. Urinalysis revealed 1+ protein, 3+ occult blood, trace of glucose. High-power field microscopic examination revealed 20 to 30 red blood cells, 8 to 10 white blood cells, 1 to 2 bacteria, 6 to 10 calcium oxalate crystals. No other abnormal findings were noted and urine was prepared for culture and sensitivity tests. The chemistry panel, including calcium and urate findings, was completely normal.

A brief nutritional assessment was obtained from Mrs. G. while her husband has having blood drawn. She indicated that her husband eats milk, ice cream, and cheese several times daily. She serves mashed potatoes with cream sauce three times a week, and he eats rhubarb, garlic, asparagus, spinach, fruit juices, chocolate milk drink (Ovaltine), beef, pork, and chicken several times a week.

STUDY QUESTIONS

1. The most likely cause of Mr. G.'s discomfort is:
   a. acute pyelonephritis
   b. cystitis
   c. urolithiasis
   d. nephrotic syndrome
   e. appendicitis

2. Which is the least likely risk factor for urolithiasis in Mr. G.?
   a. age, sex, race
   b. region of the country where he lives
   c. family history of calculi
   d. diet
   e. hyperparathyroidism

3. Further tests are ordered to determine the exact cause of Mr. G.'s disorder. Which of the following would be the most appropriate test?
   a. cystoscopy
   b. retrograde pyelography
   c. renal angiography
   d. intravenous pyelography
   e. abdominal ultrasound

4. Mr. G. is admitted for observation and therapy. In caring for him, what should the nurse recall?
   a. A lithotripter cannot be used to dislodge his kidney stone
   b. Acetaminophen (Tylenol) grains X is the pain medication most likely to be ordered
   c. Urine straining is not necessary for hospitalized individuals
   d. The individual should be taught to measure his urine pH and increase fluids

5. What would be the best urine pH for Mr. G. to maintain?
   a. neutral
   b. acid
   c. alkaline
   d. any pH

6. On IVP, Mr. G. is found to have a large staghorn calculus in the right pelvocaliceal structure. What is the most likely therapy for this gentleman?
   a. extracorporeal shock wave lithotripsy (ESWL)
   b. percutaneous nephrolithotomy (PCNL)
   c. ureterolithotomy
   d. pyelolithotomy
   e. more than one of the above

7. Which of the following is the most potentially damaging side effect of renal calculi?
   a. obstruction
   b. pain
   c. hematuria
   d. crystalluria

8. Mr. and Mrs. G. consult the dietician before discharge from the hospital. What plan would be best for him?
   a. increased yogurt, tomatoes, fluids; decreased chicken, pork, beef
   b. increased rhubarb, salmon, mutton; decreased water, oranges
   c. increased water; decreased spinach, asparagus, oranges
   d. increased parsley, garlic, rhubarb; decreased fruit juices, water

27 Acute Renal Failure

This case study will incorporate the following concepts:
1. *Glomerular filtration rate (GFR)*
2. *Sodium reabsorption*
3. *Renin mechanism*
4. *Anuria*
5. *Necrosis*
6. *Electrolyte imbalance*
7. *Metabolic acidosis*
8. *Dialysis*
9. *"Washing syndrome"*

CASE HISTORY

Mrs. S. is a 69-year-old critically ill woman who experienced a major hypotensive episode, secondary to gastrointestinal hemorrhage and hypovolemic shock.

Past History

Mrs. S. had a massive gastrointestinal bleed last night. The bleeding has stopped and she is now hemodynamically stable. However, her mean arterial pressure fell to less than 50 mm Hg for more than 40 minutes.

Current Status

Mrs. S. has no unexpected complaints. She is very relieved that her stomach ulcer has stopped bleeding. Otherwise she has only minor discomforts associated with treatment. Mrs. S.'s lying heart rate is 95 and blood pressure 138/84; standing heart rate is 100 and blood pressure 134/78. Her peripheral pulses are full (3+). She is without jugular venous distension and experiences only fleeting vertigo when sitting. Sarah has no dependent edema, her respiratory rate is 20 and unlabored, and her lungs have transitory rales that clear with coughing. Unfortunately, her urine output has been sluggish (15 to 20 ml/hr) overnight and has fallen to 10 ml/hr for the last 4 hours. The urine is a clear yellow.

Urine specific gravity is 1.010, sodium 50 mEq/L, serum blood urea nitrogen 43 mg/dl; creatinine 1.3 mg/dl. Mrs. S.'s Foley catheter irrigates easily.

STUDY QUESTIONS

1. The probable reason for a drop in GFR and subsequent oliguria while Mrs. S. was bleeding was:
   a. rapid transfusions
   b. systemic acidosis
   c. systemic hypoxia
   d. lack of renal perfusion

2. Mrs. S.'s renal renin mechanism and the release of two other hormones (aldosterone and antidiuretic hormone [ADH]) from her neuroendocrine system were called into play during her shock episode. They protected vital organs such as the brain and heart from experiencing a critical decrease in blood flow by:
   a. causing generalized vasodilatation and decreasing sodium and water resorption into the renal tubules
   b. causing secretion of dilute urine
   c. causing generalized vasoconstriction, increasing sodium and water resorption in the renal tubules, and concentrating the urine
   d. causing renal vasodilatation

Mrs. S. progresses clinically from the prerenal failure caused by shock to intrarenal failure from renal tubular cell damage. Her urine sodium level is 50 mEq/L and her specific gravity is 1.010. She appears to be normovolemic, even though her kidneys are not functioning normally.

3. Given these factors, which of the following are most helpful in monitoring Mrs. S.'s fluid states?
   a. thirst, nausea, pruritus, ecchymosis, and proteinuria
   b. blurred vision, diarrhea, pulse, and liver enlargement
   c. orthostatic changes in vital signs, edema, weight, and lung sounds
   d. orientation, arterial blood gases, heart rhythm, and coagulation studies

4. Mrs. S.'s renal renin mechanism is still active. What contribution is it making to her current state of renal damage?
   a. helping restore renal blood flow
   b. contributing to tubular necrosis by increasing ischemia
   c. maintaining normal potassium excretion
   d. assisting with sodium resorption

It is now determined that Mrs. S. has acute renal failure (ARF) caused by acute tubular necrosis (ATN). Cellular casts and epithelial debris have appeared in her urine, sloughed off by the dying tubular wall. She continues to be oliguric despite a cautious attempt to increase her renal blood flow and flush out the debris with drugs that dilate renal arteries and prevent sodium resorption in the tubules (dopamine and diuretics). Unfortunately she has no response to this treatment and it is quickly discontinued.

Two days later Mrs. S. is a little breathless, irritable, tired, and discouraged. She complains of thirst, nausea, mild pruritus (itching), weakness, and shortness of breath.

Her heart rate is 86, blood pressure 168/92, without orthostatic changes. Pulses are full (3+) and she has an S_3 heart sound (gallop). Sarah has gained 6 kg and has 3+ pitting edema around her ankles and 1+ in her knee, and sacral edema. Her lungs have fine crackles one third of the way up posteriorly. Her respiration is 24, deep and slightly labored. She is weak, lethargic, and irritable. Mrs. S.'s electrocardiogram shows tall, peaked T waves and widening intervals. Her serum blood urea nitrogen is 180 mg/dl, creatinine 10 mg/dl, potassium 7.5 mEq/L. Arterial blood pH is 7.20, $PaCO_2$ 20 mm Hg, $NaHCO_3$ 10 mEq/L, Pao_2 66 mm Hg on room air.

5. What current signs and symptoms would you attribute to Mrs. S.'s elevated potassium?
   a. electrocardiogram changes, weakness, dyspnea, irritability, and nausea
   b. pruritus, S_3 gallop, pitting edema, and weight gain
   c. thirst, hypertension, peaked T waves, oliguria, and weight gain
   d. irritability, pruritus, acidosis, S_3 gallop, weight gain, and nausea

Mrs. S. has also developed a metabolic acidosis because her kidneys cannot excrete hydrogen ions and her other compensatory mechanisms are failing.

6. What are other compensatory mechanisms of acid-base balance in Mrs. S.'s case?
   a. increased respiratory excretion of carbon dioxide (Kussmaul's respiration) and the blood buffer $NaHCO_3$
   b. Kussmaul's respiration and increasing peripheral edema
   c. blood buffer system and increasing blood urea nitrogen
   d. Kussmaul's respiration and diarrhea

Hemodialysis has become necessary. It will take care of Mrs. S.'s most urgent problems of electrolyte imbalance, acidosis, and fluid overload. Ideally dialysis will prevent additional complications of renal failure.

Ten days later, Mrs. S. is feeling better. She is able to eat, and, although her fluids are still restricted, the restriction is more liberal because of periodic dialysis.

Mrs. S.'s vital signs are closer to her normal baseline. Her edema, both peripheral and pulmonary, is gone, as are weakness and pruritus. Results of her electrocardiogram and serum electrolyte analysis are normal. Her blood urea nitrogen is 40 mg/dl and creatinine 6.0 mg/dl. Mrs. S.'s metabolic acidosis is controlled. Her urine output has increased dramatically and ranges between 100 and 150 ml/hr (2400 to 3600 ml/day).

7. Mrs. S.'s urinary output continues to be a concern because of which of the following threats?:
   a. hypervolemia and edema
   b. hypovolemia and hypokalemia
   c. hemodynamic instability and azotemia
   d. alkalosis and hypotension

Mrs. S.'s massive diuresis continued for 2 more days. Two days later she was discharged to continue recovering at home while her serum electrolytes, blood urea nitrogen, and creatinine were periodically checked. Seven months later her blood urea nitrogen plateaued at 27 mg/dl and her creatinine at 1.4 mg/dl. Mrs. S. has finally recovered.

28 Chronic Renal Failure

This case study will incorporate the following concepts:
  1. Etiology and pathology of one type of chronic renal failure
  2. Acid-base disturbance in chronic renal failure
  3. Anemia in chronic renal failure
  4. Hypertension in chronic renal failure

CASE HISTORY

Mr. B., a 35-year-old white male, was diagnosed with insulin-dependent diabetes mellitus (IDDM) in 1972 at the age of 21. He has had significant renal impairment for about 5 years and has been on a hemodialysis program for about 1 year.

Past History

Mr. B. has been on insulin since 1972. He has never been treated for ketosis or diabetic coma. His current insulin regimen is Ultra Lente, 6 units every morning and 6 units every evening, with a sliding scale of regular insulin with each meal. He has been admitted to the hospital for evaluation of his renal function and work-up for kidney transplant.

Current Status

Mr. B. states that he has gained 15 pounds over the last 3 weeks and has noted edema in both legs, which has not been significantly improved by dialysis. Blood pressure has also been elevated, measuring about 170/110. He has noted symptoms of occasional blurred vision and increasing nosebleeds. Current medications include insulin, as above, and minoxidil, 10 mg every morning and 2.5 mg every night. He has no known allergies.

His vital signs are as follows: blood pressure 190/104, heart rate 104, respirations 16, temperature 97.6° F. He has jugular venous distention without carotid bruits. Heart rhythm is regular with II/VI systolic ejection murmur at the left sternal border, no rubs noted. He has 3+ pitting edema to his knees bilaterally. Lungs are clear to auscultation and percussion bilaterally. Respiratory excursion is symmetrical and adequate bilaterally.

White blood cell count is 9600; hematocrit 31.3 ml, hemoglobin 11 g, mean corpuscular volume 88.3 μm^3, platelets 59,000/mm³, prothrombin time (PT) 9.9 sec, partial prothrombin time (PTT) 31 sec, potassium 5.2 mEq/L, sodium 134 mEq/L, glucose 228 mg/dl, blood urea nitrogen 88 mg/dl, creatinine 8.1 mg/dl, albumin 3.1 g/dl, total protein 5.5 g/dl, phosphorus 7.4 mg/dl, cholesterol 441 mg/dl, LDH 1159 units, calcium 8.9 mEq/L, pH 7.32, P_{O_2} 68 mm Hg, PCO_2 32 mm Hg, oxygen saturation 94%, bicarbonate 17 mEq/L. The urinalysis showed specific gravity of 1.009, protein 3+, blood 1+, white blood cells 5 to 6, and a few bacteria. Electrocardiogram showed a normal sinus rhythm, and chest roentgenogram indicated no acute cardiac or pulmonary pathology.

STUDY QUESTIONS

1. The morphologic changes that have occurred in Mr. B.'s diabetic neuropathy include:
   a. arteriolar sclerosis
   b. capillary basement membrane thickening
   c. nodular glomerulosclerosis
   d. all of the above

2. Mr. B.'s blood gas values suggest metabolic acidosis, reflected by his low bicarbonate and pH levels. Metabolic acidosis in chronic renal failure is due to:
   a. excess production of ammonia
   b. loss of bicarbonate in the urine
   c. loss of chloride in the urine
   d. excess retention of sulfate and phosphate

3. Mr. B.'s hemoglobin and hematocrit values are also low, indicating that he is anemic. What is the cause of this anemia accompanying his chronic renal failure?
   a. bone marrow suppression
   b. deficiency of erythropoietin
   c. shortened half-life of red blood cells
   d. increased bleeding tendency
   e. all of the above

4. Mr. B.'s blood pressure is high, measuring 190/104. Which of the following contributes most to the hypertension exprienced by most people with chronic renal failure?
   a. excess extracellular fluid volume
   b. activation of the renin-angiotensin system
   c. secretion of prostaglandins by the kidney
   d. stimulation of the renal parasympathetic nervous system
   e. a and b only

5. What does Mr. B.'s creatinine level indicate about his renal function?
   a. increasing glomerular filtration rate
   b. increasing renin production
   c. decreasing glomerular filtration rate
   d. stable excretion rates of creatinine

6. Which of the following best explains Mr. B.'s urine specific gravity of 1.009?
    a. Urinary concentration has become fixed at plasma levels as a result of severe renal failure
    b. Urinary concentration reflects adequate hydration status
    c. Urinary concentration reflects severe dehydration
    d. Urinary concentration indicates a nearly normal glomerular filtration rate

29 Surgical Ileus

This case study will incorporate the following concepts:
1. *Cause of postoperative ileus*
2. *Electrolyte imbalance*
3. *Abdominal distention*
4. *Abdominal radiographic findings*
5. *Bowel sounds*
6. *Sympathetic outflow*

CASE HISTORY

Mr. I. is a 56-year-old man admitted for elective repair of an abdominal aortic aneurysm.

Past History

Mr. I. is an active, pleasant man appearing younger than his stated age. He is a cellist in the local symphony and teaches privately in his home. He has never married. An older brother lives in town. Mr. I. has a 7-year history of adult onset diabetes and has been on insulin for the past 3 years. Past history is negative for heart or vascular disease, cancer, or pulmonary disease. Mr. I. has mild hypertension, which has been controlled with a diuretic for the last 2 years. He takes no other medications on a regular basis. Past surgical history consists of an appendectomy at age 22 and left inguinal herniorrhaphy 5 years ago.

Family history revealed that his father died of an acute myocardial infarction at age 66 and mother died of "old age" at 88 years of age. His only sibling, a 59-year-old brother, is in good health.

On routine physical examination 8 months ago, his physician noted an abdominal aortic aneurysm. Two months ago a pulsatile abdominal mass became obvious. A repeat ultrasound confirmed that the aneurysm was enlarging. A referral was made to a vascular surgeon, who recommended repair. Mr. I. was admitted to the general surgical ward, where he had preoperative tests and teaching in preparation for surgery.

Current Status

After 10 hours of uncomplicated surgery Mr. I. was transferred to the surgical intensive care unit. On arrival he was awake though drowsy from the morphine sulfate that he was receiving every 1 1/2 to 2 hours for pain. His skin was flushed, warm, and dry. A nitroprusside drip was infusing at 1.2 μm/kg/min to maintain his systolic blood pressure at less than 160. His heart rate remained in the 90s and his respiratory rate was 22 on 40% oxygen through a face mask. His hematocrit remained stable at 38% for last 5 hours. His abdomen was moderately distended, but soft, with no bowel sounds heard after a prolonged period of auscultation. A nasogastric tube was positioned and connected to low constant suction to ensure gastric decompression.

On the first postoperative day his abdominal girth was 86.2 cm. Nasogastric output was measured every 4 hours and fluctuated from 75 to 200 cc of light green drainage. Antacid/antiflatulent (Mylanta) 30 ml was administered through the nasogastric tube every 2 hours because his gastric pH was running less than 5.0. The nasogastric tube was clamped from suction for 30 minutes after each dose. In addition to the usual intravenous therapy for fluid maintenance, his nasogastric output was replaced milliliter for milliliter with D_5•45 normal saline (NS) and potassium chloride (KCl) 20 mEq/L.

STUDY QUESTIONS

1. According to recent research, which of the following was most likely the cause of Mr. I.'s ileus?
   a. opiates
   b. anesthetic agents
   c. surgical manipulation of bowel
   d. sympathetic nervous system mediated reflex

2. Which of the following *does not* inhibit postoperative ileus resolution?
   a. hypokalemia
   b. peritonitis
   c. duration of surgery
   d. retroperitoneal extravasation of fluids

3. Mr. I. received potassium chloride (KCl) because an ileus can produce which one of the following lab pictures?:
   a. hypokalemia
   b. hyponatremia
   c. alkalosis (respiratory) and metabolic acidosis
   d. alkalosis (metabolic) and respiratory acidosis

On the second postoperative day, nitroprusside dosage was tapered and then discontinued as intravenous methyldopa (Aldomet) was able to control his hypertension. He was placed on 3 L of oxygen after demonstrating adequate oxygenation. Analgesia was being maintained with morphine 8 mg intramuscularly every 4 hours. His abdomen was only mildly distended and soft with bowel sounds audible in all four quadrants. A decision was made to leave his nasogastric tube in place until morning.

On the third postoperative day his abdominal girth was 82.8 cm, a decrease of 3.4 cm from postoperative day 1. Nasogastric output was slowed to 100 ml every 8 hours. He did not require antacid/antiflatulent (Mylanta) and tolerated his nasogastric tube clamped for 2 hours with residuals of 50 ml. His gastric output continued to be replaced milliliter for milliliter with $D_5 \cdot 45$ NS + 20 mEq KCl. He remained on "nothing by mouth" status and was encouraged to brush his teeth every 4 to 6 hours.

4. Which of the following signs will *best* indicate a return to adequate bowel function for Mr. I.?
   a. complaints of hunger
   b. presence of bowel sounds
   c. flatus and/or stool passed
   d. minimal gastric output

Mr. I. was transferred to the surgical ward on his fourth postoperative day. His nasogastric tube was removed, and he was taking a clear liquid diet well this morning. At about 10:00 a.m. he began to complain of increasing abdominal discomfort, and feeling "bloated", he was nauseated and had one episode of vomiting 200 ml of light green fluid. His respiratory rate increased to 30 breaths/min on 3 L of oxygen. His heart rate increased from 94 to 110/min. His blood pressure and temperature were normal.

A nasogastric tube was passed with an immediate return of 300 ml light green stomach contents. Abdominal girth was 85 cm. Bowel sounds, which had been active in the morning, were absent. An emergency erect abdominal roentgenogram revealed the presence of scattered air/fluid levels. A follow-up film 3 hours later showed little change in the air/fluid distribution. Bowel sounds returned slowly the next morning and a diagnosis of recurrent ileus over obstruction was made.

5. Which one of these factors would *not* have contributed to the recurrence of Mr. I.'s ileus?
   a. resumption of oral intake
   b. electrolyte, especially potassium, imbalance
   c. diabetes
   d. hypertension

6. Which of the following *is not* a typical clinical feature of ileus in Mr. I.?
   a. abdominal film demonstrating a local loop of dilated small bowel in the absence of gas in the colon
   b. presence of gas and fluid together, possibly allowing a splash to be elicited
   c. absence of bowel sounds
   d. tachypnea

7. Which one of the following treatments would be contraindicated in treating Mr. I.?
   a. enemas/cathartics
   b. gastric decompression
   c. analgesics

30 Peptic Ulcer Disease

This case study will incorporate the following concepts:
  1. Differentiation of gastric and duodenal ulcers
  2. Risk factors and cause of ulcers
  3. Common complications of ulcers
  4. Physiological changes and common complications resulting from surgical inter-
     ventions for ulcer disease (Billroth I and II)

CASE HISTORY

Ms. K. is a 44-year-old white female who was admitted for diagnostic work-up of persistent abdominal pain. She is the mother of three young children (ages 10, 8, and 6); she is employed in a management position with an advertising agency and works long hours. Her husband died this past year.

Past History

Karen has a history of smoking 1 pack/day of cigarettes. Her eating habits are irregular, and she frequently takes aspirin for mild headaches. Having been diagnosed with rheumatoid arthritis 2 years ago, Karen takes 10 mg/day of prednisone. Family history revealed that her father has complained of "gastritis-like" symptoms for the last 10 years, although he has never tested for this problem. The remaining history was unremarkable except for incidences of hypertension in a paternal uncle and a maternal grandmother.

Current Status

Ms. K. is 5 feet 3 inches and currently weighs 100 pounds, having lost 10 pounds during the last 6 weeks. Blood pressure on admission was 150/88. For the last 3 months she has been experiencing mild intermittent epigastric pain. The week before admission the pain became more continuous, becoming intense 1 to 2 hours after eating. Eating occasionally relieves the pain temporarily. She also experienced slight nausea throughout the last week with one episode of hematemesis the evening before admission.

On admission, Ms. K. was kept on "nothing by mouth" status. A nasogastric tube was inserted and connected to intermittent suction, and intravenous fluid replacement begun. Cimetidine was given intravenously and antacids were administered through a nasogastric tube. Ms. K. experienced a massive upper gastrointestinal bleed 2 days after admission. Treatment included iced saline nasogastric irrigations, intravenous pitressin tannate, and blood transfusions. In 24 hours she had a recurrence of bleeding bright red blood through the nasogastric tube and her rectum. Gastroscopy indicated gastric and pyloric ulcers, hemoglobin 7.8 g, hematocrit 21%. Billroth II (hemigastrectomy and gastrojejunostomy with vagotomy) surgery was performed.

Ten days post surgery Ms. K. started on a bland diet. Almost immediately after meals, she began to experience epigastric fullness, distention, discomfort, abdominal cramping, nausea, and flatus.

STUDY QUESTIONS

1. In Ms. K.'s case, what contributing factors would be relevant to her developing a peptic ulcer disease?
   a. smoking
   b. ingesting anti-inflammatory agents
   c. hereditary factors
   d. all of the above

2. Before admission Ms. K. experienced a great deal of abdominal discomfort about 1 to 2 hours after eating. The underlying physiological reason for this is:
   a. edematous duodenum resulting from the mechanical pressure placed on it by the semidigested meal
   b. increased back-diffusion of ingested acid into the mucosa
   c. increased gastrin concentration in the antral mucosa caused by the ingestion of proteins

3. You will be assessing Ms. K. for signs and symptoms related to which of the following most frequent complications of peptic ulcer disease?
   a. gastric outlet obstruction
   b. hemorrhage
   c. anemia
   d. perforation
   e. a, c
   f. b, c
   g. a, d
   h. a, b, d

4. The symptoms that Ms. K. experienced 10 days after surgery are suggestive of what postsurgical complication?
   a. dumping syndrome
   b. surgical ileus
   c. metabolic acidosis
   d. fistula

5. Approximately 2 weeks after Karen is discharged home, she returns to the clinic complaining of epigastric fullness after eating that is relieved by vomiting. She also has intermittent abdominal pain. Symptoms suggest:
   a. reflux gastritis
   b. afferent loop obstruction
   c. muscle spasms
   d. surgical stress ulcer

31 Alcoholic Cirrhosis

This case study will incorporate the following concepts:
1. *Mechanisms of ascites and edema*
2. *Portal hypertension*
3. *Liver dysfunction*
4. *Chronic hepatic portosystemic encephalopathy*

CASE HISTORY

Mr. S., a 50-year-old man, has been admitted to the hospital for treatment of acute gastrointestinal bleed. He is well known to the medical community for his chronic alcohol abuse and encephalopathy.

Past History

Mr. S. has been hospitalized four times in the past 24 months; most recently he was discharged 12 weeks ago for treatment of upper gastrointestinal bleeding. He has a 40-year history of smoking and drinks an unknown quantity of liquor daily. On previous admissions he has been treated for pancreatitis, alcohol withdrawal seizures, cirrhosis and associated ascites, coagulopathy, esophageal varices, anemia, gastrointestinal bleed, and gastritis.

Current Status

His current problems include hepatic encephalopathy, gastrointestinal bleed, coagulopathy, jaundice, history of tuberculosis (age 15 with treatment), and hypoxia; all present were on previous admission. Medications at last discharge included spironolactone (25 mg twice a day), ranitidine (150 mg twice a day), antacid (Maalox), and multivitamins.

Mr. S. was found unconscious in a pool of blood and vomitus. He was taken to the hospital and admitted to the medical intensive care unit. Initial vital signs were as follows: blood pressure 90/60, heart rate 112, respirations 12. Intravenous infusion with normal saline was begun through a central line; oxygen was started at 3 L by nasal cannula. Physical examination revealed icteric sclera, clear lungs, grade III/IV systolic ejection murmur, abdomen soft and without masses, liver percussed at 12 cm below the costal margin, and skin markedly jaundiced. Deep tendon reflexes were brisk and equal bilaterally.

Lab tests revealed the following: sodium 137 mEq/L, potassium 4.8 mEq/L, chloride 102 mEq/L, carbon dioxide 23 mEq/L, blood urea nitrogen 132 mg/dl, creatinine 1.3 mg/dl, glucose 115 mg/dl, hematocrit 27.7%, hemoglobin 9.3 g, white blood cell count 17,800 mm³, platelets 259,000 mm³, direct bilirubin 7.8 mg/dl, total bilirubin 16.4 mg/dl, amylase 42 somogyi units/dl, alkaline phosphatase 127 mu/dl, ammonia level 200 mg. Blood gases were as follows: Po_2 85 mm Hg, PCO_2 30 mm Hg, pH 7.35, prothrombin time (PT) patient 17 sec, prothrombin time (PT) control 12.3 sec, partial prothrombin time (PTT) 46/36 sec.

Treatment with blood replacement was initiated; it included transfusion of 6 units fresh frozen plasma and 5 units packed red blood cells, with antacids, ranitidine, vitamin K, thiamine, and lactulose by nasogastric tube.

On the following day Mr. S.'s mental status was improved and his laboratory studies were as follows: sodium 133 mEq/L, potassium 3.5 mEq/L, chloride 105 mEq/L, blood urea nitrogen 15 mg/dl, creatinine 0.7 mg/dl, glucose 114 mg/dl, hematocrit 38.7%, white blood cell count 5200 mm³, PT 15.7/12 sec, ammonia 93 mg, alkaline phosphatase 92 μ/dl. Vital signs were as follows: blood pressure 116/72, heart rate 72, respirations 15, afebrile.

On day 2 he was oriented X3 and was transferred from the intensive care unit. During the course of his hospitalization his total bilirubin ranged from 16.4 mg/dl down to 10.7 mg/dl at discharge.

STUDY QUESTIONS

1. Mr. S.'s observed electrolyte imbalances were caused by which of the following?:
   a. jaundice
   b. ascites and edema
   c. hyperalbuminemia

2. One of the major complications of cirrhosis that can ultimately lead to massive hemorrhage and death for Mr. S. is:
   a. esophageal varices
   b. infection
   c. poor nutritional intake

3. Mr. S.'s decreased level of consciousness was caused by:
   a. blood loss
   b. jaundice
   c. hepatic encephalopathy

4. Mr. S. was exhibiting coagulopathies caused by which of the following mechanisms:
   a. collection of blood in the gut
   b. interruption of normal clotting mechanisms
   c. hemolytic reaction to blood transfusion

CASE STUDY 32 Gastroenteritis with Dehydration

This case study will incorporate the following concepts:
1. *Body fluids and electrolytes in infants and children*
2. *Parenteral fluid therapy*
3. *Infant nutrition*
4. *Alterations in hydrogen ion concentration*

CASE HISTORY

K.L. was a 7-week-old infant who was taken to the emergency room of a local hospital because her parents were concerned about vomiting and diarrhea.

Past History

Three days before admission K.L. began to have frequent, watery stools, 8 to 10/day. She was irritable, cried for long periods of time, and had a rectal temperature of 38.4° C. During the first day of illness, she continued to take normal feedings of infant formula (Similac 20), but by the second day her appetite had decreased and she began taking only small amounts of weak tea with sugar. During the 12 hours before admission K.L. had 8 watery stools.

The following were significant physical findings: K.L. was lethargic but arousable with stimulation; muscle tone was weak; K.L. displayed no muscle twitching or irritability; anterior fontanel was depressed; eyes appeared sunken and had dark circles around them; no tears were present. Skin in general was cool and gray; abdominal skin showed loss of elasticity (skin remained in folds when pinched). Peripheral pulses were weak; capillary refill time was 3 to 4 seconds. Rectal temperature was 36.2° C, heart rate 176, blood pressure 90/58, and respirations 56. Weight 3 kg, length 49 cm, head circumference 35 cm.

Current Status

K.L. was admitted to the hospital for treatment of gastroenteritis with dehydration.

Clinical signs indicated that she had lost approximately 10% of her body weight because of lost fluids. An intravenous catheter was inserted, and the following fluids and volumes were infused: 60 ml fresh frozen plasma was given within a 20-minute period; 60 ml $D_{10}W$ was given over 20 minutes; 40 mEq/L D_5W with sodium, 20 mEq/L potassium, 40 mEq/L chloride. Base 20 mEq/L was given at a rate of 26 ml/hr for 7 hours. D_5W with the preceding electrolytes was given at 19 ml/hr for 16 hours, and all ongoing fluid losses from emesis and bowel movements were replaced milliliter for milliliter. No oral fluids were given during the first 24 hours of hospitalization. The infant was placed in isolation to prevent spread of possible infectious organisms to other patients or personnel.

The following laboratory studies were performed: arterial blood gases, serum electrolytes, complete blood count, blood urea nitrogen, creatinine, and stool culture and antibiotic sensitivity tests. The results of the laboratory studies were within normal limits except for the following arterial blood gases: pH 7.28, Po_2 96 mm Hg, PCO_2 22 mm Hg, bicarbonate 9 mEq/L, base excess −15. Electrolytes were as follows: sodium 136 mEq/L, chloride 114 mEq/L, potassium 4.2 mEq/L, bicarbonate 9 mEq/L. Urine specific gravity was 1.020. K.L. improved rapidly after infusion of the plasma and $D_{10}W$. She became more alert and active. Her heart rate decreased to 124, respirations to 42, blood pressure to 90/50. She voided 15 ml urine.

On the second hospital day oral feedings of oral electrolyte solution (Pedialyte) were tolerated well. One-fourth strength infant formula without lactose and with predigested protein (Pregestimil) was introduced. The intravenous D_5W with electrolytes was discontinued after determination that oral intake was sufficient to maintain adequate fluid volume. Her total fluid intake was 140 ml/kg/day, or 420 ml. The urine output was 210 ml and stool output was 15 ml.

K.L. was discharged from the hospital on the third hospital day. Her parents were instructed to continue oral feedings. The infant was seen in the outpatient clinic on the seventh day after her hospital admission. She was taking infant formula (Similac 20) 15 ounces/24 hr) without diarrhea. She weighed 3.5 kg. Findings of a physical examination were within normal limits. The cause of the acute diarrheal disturbance was diagnosed as viral gastroenteritis, and she recovered well from the effects of the illness and accompanying dehydration and acidosis.

STUDY QUESTIONS

1. Which of the following factors contributes most to the infant's vulnerability to altered fluid/electrolyte balance?
   a. Sixty percent of the total body weight in infants is water
   b. The infant's metabolic rate is lower than the adult's
   c. The infant normally loses and replaces 25% of the total body water in 24 hours
   d. The infant's body is composed of a greater proportion of fat than the adult's

2. A useful physical sign in evaluating fluid deficits in infants is:
   a. hyperthermia
   b. decreased peripheral perfusion
   c. irritability
   d. hyperventilation

3. Which of the following best explains the cause of K.L.'s diarrhea on the first day of her illness?
   a. Irritation of the gastrointestinal tract causes increased intestinal motility
   b. The infectious agent invades the gastrointestinal mucosa and alters the balance of water and electrolytes
   c. Secondary lactose intolerance from the milk-based formula alters fluid balance
   d. "Starvation diarrhea" results when formula and clear fluids are the only source of nutrition

4. The immediate goal of rapid infusion of intravenous fluids during the initial treatment of dehydration is to replace fluid in which of the following compartments?
   a. intracellular
   b. intravascular
   c. transcellular
   d. all body fluid compartments

5. Vomiting and diarrhea cause hydrogen ion disturbances by which of the following mechanisms?
   a. loss of bicarbonate as a result of vomiting
   b. catabolism of glycogen in the liver
   c. loss of hydrogen ion in the urine
   d. lactic acid production secondary to decreased perfusion

6. Which factor most likely caused the change in K.L.'s potassium level?
   a. acidosis
   b. alkalosis
   c. intravenous infusion of calcium
   d. intravenous infusion of glucose

7. On the basis of K.L.'s electrolyte levels, which of the following is the type of dehydration she had?
   a. isonatremic
   b. hyponatremic
   c. hypernatremic

33 Degenerative Joint Disease

This case study incorporates the following concepts:
1. *Etiology of osteoporosis*
2. *Pathophysiology of osteoporosis*
3. *Cartilage erosion*
4. *Osteophyte formation*

CASE HISTORY

Past History

At age 10 Mr. D. had a developmental disorder of the epiphyseal ossification center. The disorder was treated conservatively with crutches and an ischial weight-bearing brace. He remained active over subsequent years with intermittent mild discomfort. At age 20 he noticed increasing pain during activities such as golf and jogging. Since then the pain has become increasingly worse in the hip and groin. He also reports clicking, popping, and giving way of his right hip. For the past 4 years he has ambulated with a cane. Two months ago he fell, severely aggravating his pain, and he now requires crutches for walking.

Current Status

Extremities: the lower left extremity appears 0.5 cm shorter than the right; there is no sign of skin changes around the right or left hip. Range of motion: left hip flexion is normal; abduction is 40 degrees, internal rotation 40 degrees, extension full, adduction 40 degrees, external rotation 40 degrees; right hip flexion is 100 degrees; abduction 20 degrees; internal rotation 30 degrees, extension full, adduction 15 degrees, external rotation 0 degrees. Anterior-posterior roentgenogram of the right hip shows extensive changes with aseptic necrosis and deformity of the right femoral head. The femoral head is oblong with loose cartilaginous fragments and osteophytes. Cystic areas and sclerosis are prominent in the upper one third of the right femur.

STUDY QUESTIONS

1. Given Mr. D.'s history, which type of degenerative joint disease does he have?
   a. primary
   b. inflammatory
   c. secondary
   d. traumatic

2. What pathophysiological change in the right hip subjects the femoral head to cyst formation?
   a. erosion of cartilage
   b. osteophyte formation
   c. loss of proprioceptive reflexes
   d. skeletal deformity

3. Which of the following pathophysiological changes is/are characteristic of degenerative joint disease?
   a. elongated femoral femur and osteophytes
   b. septic necrosis
   c. sclerosis of the femur and osteophytes
   d. shortened extremity
   e. all of the above

4. Which of the clinical findings are definitely related to Mr. D.'s current complaint of pain?
   a. loose cartilaginous fragments and cyst formation
   b. osteophyte and cyst formations
   c. cyst formation and limited range of motion
   d. all of the above

5. Mr. D. reports that his right hip gives way, which indicates that he may also have:
   a. damage to the joint's supporting structure
   b. an underlying neurological disorder
   c. chronic inflammation in the joint
   d. damage to the synovial lining

6. Physical examination reveals limited range of motion in Mr. D.'s right hip. What is the primary cause of his limited range of motion?
   a. osteophyte fragments
   b. loss of proprioceptive reflexes
   c. formation of new bone
   d. degeneration of articular cartilage

34 Rheumatoid Arthritis

This case study will incorporate the following concepts:
1. *Articular cartilage destruction*
2. *Etiology of rheumatoid arthritis*
3. *Lysosomal enzymes*

CASE HISTORY

Mrs. O. is a 52-year-old homemaker with a 15-year history of rheumatoid arthritis.

Past History

Over the years Mrs. O. has undergone many treatment modalities, but her disease has been unresponsive. Six months ago she experienced a generalized flare-up of acute arthritis that involved her shoulders, knees, hands, and feet. During the past year she has experienced increasingly severe pain and stiffness in her left hip. The pain persists at rest and severely limits her activity and weight bearing. She has difficulty walking, using stairs, getting up from a chair, putting on shoes and socks, dressing, bathing, and sitting up from a supine position. She is steroid-dependent on 1 mg of prednisone and is generally confined to a wheelchair.

Current Status

Mrs. O. has marked deformities of both hands, ulnar subluxation of the metacarpophalangeal joints and boutonnière and swan neck deformities. She has limited range of motion in the left hip but no tenderness on palpation. Her gait is labored, very slow, and shuffling.

Range of motion: left hip flexion 75%, extension full external rotation 0 degrees, internal rotation 5 degrees; right hip flexion 120 degrees, extension full external rotation 3 degrees, internal rotation 30 degrees. Roentgenogram of the left hip reveals absent or markedly thin articular cartilage along the articular surface of the joint. The femoral head reveals a moderate degree of inflammatory infiltration, fibrosis, and sclerosis.

1. Which one of the following pathophysiological changes most likely accounts for Mrs. O.'s inability to rise from a chair or a supine position?
   a. synovial edema
   b. joint rupture
   c. pannus formation
   d. articular cartilage destruction

2. Which of the following statements explains Mrs. O.'s generalized flare-up of rheumatoid arthritis?
   a. exposure to influenza virus
   b. increased production of rheumatoid factor
   c. systemic nature of the disease
   d. increased levels of immunoglobulin G (IgG)

3. What physiological mechanism is directly responsible for the marked absence of articular cartilage seen on Mrs. O.'s roentgenogram?
   a. immune complex formation
   b. lysosomal degradation
   c. antigen-antibody formation
   d. lymphocyte response

4. What is the rationale for instituting range of motion exercises for Mrs. O.?
   a. preventing decreased activity, which can result in muscle atrophy
   b. slowing the inflammatory response
   c. increasing formation of lymphocytes
   d. preventing synovial joint ruptures

5. Which complication must Mrs. O. become aware of?
   a. bone marrow destruction
   b. flexion of involved joints
   c. formation of cysts
   d. elongation of ligaments

6. What is the primary reason for treating Mrs. O. with the steroid prednisone?
   a. to combat the inflammatory response activated by immune complexes
   b. to combat pannus formation activated by cartilage destruction
   c. to alleviate her pain and stiffness symptoms
   d. to prevent further loss of mobility

This case study will incorporate the following concepts:

1. *Etiology of burns*
2. *Evaluation of burn injury severity*
   a. *Depth*
   b. *Extent*
   c. *Physiology of tissue injury*
   d. *Burn shock*
   1) *Electrolyte balance*
   2) *Fluid loss*
3. *Special care area*
   a. *Circumferential burns*
4. *Fluid resuscitation*
5. *Nutrition*
   a. *Hypermetabolism*
   b. *Protein wasting*

CASE HISTORY

Mr. B. is a 32-year-old Caucasian male who has sustained a 58% total body surface area (TBSA) burn as the result of an indoor explosion in the sawmill where he is employed.

Past History

Mr. B. is a well-nourished, slender male who has been healthy until this event. He does not smoke but reports drinking one case of beer a week for the last 5 years. He has never been seriously ill nor had any operations. Mr. B. is married and the father of two healthy children. His family history indicates no hypertension, diabetes, or heart, lung, or kidney disease.

Current Status

Mr. B. was air-lifted to the regional burn trauma center about 4 hours after the explosion. The referring local hospital had initially stabilized Mr. B. by intubating him, starting intravenous therapy, placing a catheter into his bladder, inserting a nasogastric tube, and performing bilateral upper extremity escharotomies (removal of eschar).

On admission to the burn unit initial assessment revealed that Mr. B. received a 58% TBSA (see the figure below). He was observed to have full thickness burns on his face, bilaterally and circumferentially to both arms, and bilaterally to the dorsal areas of his hands and burn patches to both posterior surfaces of the thighs (accounting for 40% of TBSA). These burn areas were dry, hard, and leathery in appearance. He stated that these areas were not painful when touched or exposed to the air. The remaining 18% of TBSA demonstrated second-degree burns. These areas included burns to the posterior of the head and back of neck, buttocks, and palms and to the anterior portion of the thighs. These wounds were red in appearance with serous fluid seeping from many open areas. Thin-walled blisters were formed in these areas, causing him a great deal of pain.

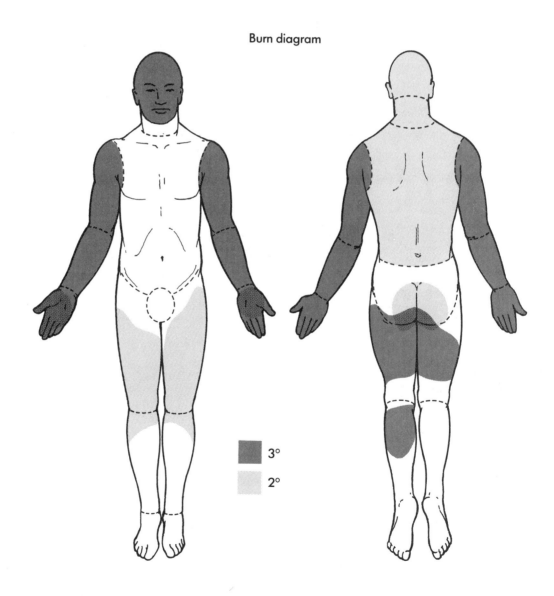

Burn diagram

3°

2°

Mr. B. had received 6000 ml of Ringer's lactate by the time of admission to the burn unit. His output was maintained at approximately 30 ml/hr since catheterization.

Further evaluation revealed that Mr. B. was developing periorbital edema. His pharynx and chest were clear to auscultation. Respirations were at 22, unlabored. Cardiac status revealed a regular heart rate with no ectopic beats or sounds. There was marked swelling and tightness of the skin on both arms and hands. Mr. B. was alert and oriented to his surroundings.

Initial laboratory values were as follows: white blood count 20,000 mm^3, hematocrit 45.5%, sodium 120 mEq/L, potassium 3.4 mEq/L, chloride 101 mEq/L, bicarbonate 24 mEq/L, blood urea nitrogen 17 mg/dl, glucose 244 mg/dl. Initial vital signs were as follows: blood pressure (lying) 124/78, heart rate 128, respirations 22, rectal temperature 38.5° C.

Fluid resuscitation was accomplished in the first 24 hours after the burn by using the Parkland fluid resuscitation formula. On the basis of body weight and burn area, it was calculated that Mr. B. required 22,772 ml (5 ml/kg weight × %TBSA) of Ringer's lactate to regain his capillary seal.

Burn treatment consisted of cleansing the areas three times a day with cleanser (Hibiclens). This was followed by application of antibiotic (Bacitracin) to his face, antibiotic (Sulfamylon Acetate Cream) to his ears, and 1% silver Sulfadiazine (Silvadene) to his trunk and extremities. A light dressing (Kerlix) was applied. Mr. B. began Hubbard tank treatments on postburn day 4. All of his hair was shaved daily within 2 inches of his burns. His nutritional needs were calculated at 412 k cal/day to achieve a positive nitrogen balance. Mr. B. received three high-protein, high-calorie meals a day. This nutritional intake was supplemented with enteral feedings delivered at 170 ml/hr for 47 days.

Excision and grafting procedures were begun on postburn day 9 on the upper extremities. On postburn days 23 and 24 he underwent excision and grafting procedures to the face. A bilateral tarsorrhaphy was performed to correct for developing ectropion (eversion of eyelid edges). Mr. B. had 100% adherence and viability of all skin grafts.

Physical therapy began on the day of admission and he was ambulated on postburn day 7. At this time he was started on a concentrated exercise program that involved specific routines as well as active range of motion. Mr. B. was expected also to perform all activities of daily living.

STUDY QUESTIONS

1. Burn shock can best be described as:
   a. hypovolemic shock
   b. cardiogenic shock
   c. septic shock
   d. neurogenic shock

2. Which of the following most likely accounts for Mr. B.'s initial need for nasotracheal intubation?
   a. burned lungs
   b. facial edema
   c. extent and depth of neck burn
   d. fluid overload

3. Mr. B.'s initial hematocrit was 45.41 ml. What physiological phenomenon is most likely accounting for this elevation?
   a. increased demand of the burned tissue for oxygen
   b. leakage of intracellular fluids from the capillaries
   c. decreased fluid intake over the past 24 hours
   d. hemostatic reaction to the inflammatory process

4. Escharotomy, a cut through circumferential area of burned skin, was performed for the purpose of:
   a. decreasing the effects of hypovolemia
   b. preventing infection to the extremities
   c. checking the depth of the burns
   d. restoring adequate blood supply to the distal areas

5. Mr. B. complains of a great deal of pain in areas where he received second-degree burns, but not in the area of the more extensive third-degree burns. The best explanation for this phenomenon is that:
   a. In third-degree burns the dermis has been destroyed
   b. Eschar formation in areas of third-degree burns acts as a protection for the exposed nerve endings
   c. Vesiculation in areas of second-degree burns continually irritates the exposed nerve endings
   d. Mr. B. suffered more second-degree burns, and his pain is related to the size of the burn area

6. Lactated Ringer's solution was chosen for the resuscitation phase of burn treatment for Mr. B. The physiological rationale for this choice is that:
   a. Ringer's lactate is high in sodium and slows the loss of intracellular fluid by increasing the serum osmolality
   b. Ringer's lactate closely resembles extracellular fluid in composition and helps rapidly replace the fluid being lost from the extracellular compartments
   c. Ringer's lactate is able to replace the amount of plasma being lost by encouraging the metabolism of protein
   d. Lactated Ringer's solution increases the hydrostatic pressure in the extracellular spaces, creating a transverse fluid gradient

7. When Mr. B. started his hydrotherapy treatments, his nurse was very careful to limit his time in the tank to 30 minutes. She needed to be so fastidious about the time because:
   a. The skin around the burn areas is very friable and as a result easily breaks down
   b. The skin around the burn areas will shrink, causing strictures in a short period of time
   c. The sodium loss resulting from the hydrotherapy must be minimized as much as possible
   d. Excessive exposure to warm water makes individuals with burns hypotensive

8. The nurses noted that on the initial history and physical examination in the burn unit Mr. B. had an absence of bowel sounds. The best explanation for this finding is that:
   a. He has some underlying intestinal problems that were precipitated by the burn trauma
   b. He has had no food for the last 6 hours
   c. His intestinal mucosa has become edematous as the result of the burn trauma
   d. He is beginning to present with signs of hypovolemic shock

9. Mr. B. was sent home with Jobst stockings along with instructions to wear them for 1 year. When he questions the need for this, you explain that:
   a. A gentle constant pressure should be applied to the newly grafted areas for approximately 1 year to promote circulation
   b. Skin grafts must be protected from any kind of trauma for at least 1 year; Jobsts provide a layer of protection against such external insult
   c. The consistent application of Jobsts will prevent hyperpigmentation, which leads to greater scarring
   d. The Jobsts serve as a protection against the effects of ultraviolet radiation on the new graft sites

ANSWERS WITH RATIONALES

1 Trisomy 21/Down syndrome

1. **c** that these characteristics are most properly related to some sort of chromosomal defect

   Rationale
   Neither parental morning sickness, unusual presentations during delivery, nor cord trauma is known to produce the physical characteristics seen in this baby. These findings represent abnormal fetal development and are very likely due to a genetic malformation. In this particular syndrome, the newborn often is "floppy," has a flat occiput, and is short, in addition to the findings described in the case.

2. **a** These two findings are called epicanthal folds and simian creases, respectively; these findings are seen in approximately 50% of all babies born with trisomy 21

   Rationale
   Epicanthal folds and simian creases are characteristic of trisomy 21. If present at birth, they are often the first indicators that a genetic defect is present. Although these same features occur in the general population approximately 5% to 20% of the time, it would be inappropriate to lead Mrs. H. to believe that her baby is normal. Features that are the result of genetic aberration are permanent.

3. **c** analyzing the chromosomal formation of his white blood cells

   Rationale
   The term *phenotype* refers to the physical appearance or makeup of the individual and does not reveal the source of aberration. *Barr bodies* are part of the sex chromatin mass, and trisomy 21 is an autosomal aberration. Although it would be helpful to establish chromosomal patterns in both parents in cases where inheritance may be a factor, in the majority of cases of Down syndrome in older women the aberration is not linked to parental chromosomal patterns.

4. **d** failure of two chromosomes to separate during the first meiotic phase of cellular division

Rationale
Nondisjunction occurs in meiosis during anaphase I or II, or in the anaphase of mitosis. Simply stated, it is the failure of chromosomes to separate. Nondisjunction is the most frequent accident involving the whole chromosome. It accounts for approximately 85% of all trisomy 21 cases and is the most common underlying cause of Down syndrome in babies born to older women.

5. **c** Down syndrome occurs when the chromosomes fail to divide properly, usually as a result of multiple factors

Rationale
Down syndrome occurs when the twenty-first chromosome fails to divide properly, creating a trisomic condition. The cause of this chromosomal aberration is multifactoral, having been attributed to genetic predisposition, environmental factors, and chance occurrences. The majority of cases are due to nondisjunction, and of these, 75% arise from nondisjunction of the mother's cells and 25% from the father's cells. About 4% of Down syndrome cases are caused by translocation of the twenty-first chromosome. This defect is hereditary and is not associated with parental age, as in nondisjunction. Approximately 1% of Down syndrome cases result from mosaicism, which is a partial trisomy caused by an error in very early cell division. The risk of having a baby with Down syndrome for a mother who is 45 years or older is about 1 in 16, or 6%. As stated previously, these cases usually result from nondisjunction. Chromosomal analysis can determine which of these abnormalities exists and can help predict the risk to a given set of parents of producing another Down syndrome child.

6. **b** Metabolic and enzyme functions are frequently altered in Down syndrome babies

Rationale
In Down syndrome, metabolic processes and enzyme factors may be altered. This alteration is caused by the triplication of the genes governing these functions. Nurses caring for babies with trisomy 21 must be aware that gastrointestinal complications, particularly intestinal atresia, are frequent.

7. **d** Babies with Down syndrome often have cardiac anomalies, respiratory infections, kidney problems, and tracheoesophageal fistulae.

Rationale
Babies with Down syndrome are at risk for several functional abnormalities that have been well described in the literature. About 40% to 50% have congenital heart disease, especially septal defects. Other structural defects, such as intestinal atresia, renal agenesis, and tracheoesophageal fistula, are also common. Although the exact mechanisms for these structural problems are not clear, they all represent an interruption or alteration in normal fetal development. Children with Down syndrome are also at risk for increased respiratory infections. It is postulated that hypotonic chest muscles may contribute to an increased susceptibility to these infections. In fact, the combination of congenital heart disease and respiratory illness is the main cause of death in children with Down syndrome who die in the first year of life.

8. **a** Every child with Down syndrome has some degree of mental retardation but most have IQs within the "trainable" range

Rationale
It is true that one of the main features of Down syndrome is some degree of mental retardation. Though the mean (average) IQs for people with Down syndrome are 41.7 for males and 49.9 for females, it is also true that about 40% of these children have IQs greater than 50. In any case, these children's developmental delays represent a major challenge for parents and communities. Parents should know that development will have peaks and plateaus and that motor development may lag behind mental development. Though it was very common to institutionalize such children in the past, it is now felt that most parents can provide the environment necessary for optimal development and health in the home.

2 Wound Healing

1. **a** Inflammation

   Rationale

   Inflammation is one of the initial processes of normal wound healing. Failure of the inflammatory response predisposes the wound to infection, which inhibits all other processes of healing. The diabetic may fail to mount a sufficient inflammatory response in relation to wound healing because of leukocyte dysfunction. Without sufficient insulin to facilitate transfer of glucose into the leukocytes, these cells fail to receive the energy needed for chemotaxis, phagocytosis, and intracellular killing. These leukocyte functions are important in the prevention of infection. Although Mrs. P. had been taking her insulin as prescribed, during periods of physiological stress (such as that associated with wounding) blood glucose levels are higher than usual. Under these conditions, additional insulin is required to transport glucose into the cell. It is also essential that the wound receive sufficient nutrients to support the energy depleting activities of inflammation; among these nutrients is oxygen. The small vessel disease associated with diabetes that was evident in Mrs. P.'s extremities would impair oxygen delivery to the heel wound.

2. **b** secondary intention

Rationale

Mrs. P.'s heel wound was "crater-like" in appearance when she sought medical care. This indicates that a large amount of tissue destruction had taken place. Before the completion of healing, destroyed tissue must be replaced in the open wound bed. This occurs mainly through the processes of epithelialization, collagen metabolism, and contraction. Wounds that heal by replacement of lost tissue are said to heal by secondary intention, in contrast to healing by primary intention, which occurs in surgically created wounds. In these wounds, a surgically created incision is sutured together and thus tissue loss is minimized. The processes of epithelialization and contraction are not as pronounced in these wounds. Before healing by second intention, necrotic tissue must be cleared from the wound bed to enable the migration of healthy new epithelial cells. This is the rationale behind the debriding by saline-soaked kerlix.

3. **b** hypoxemia

Rationale

When a wound becomes infected, there will be prolongation of the inflammatory response in an attempt to fight the infection. Therefore, among the signs and symptoms associated with infection will be those associated with inflammation. These would include the classic signs of inflammation: redness, heat, pain, swelling, and loss of function. In addition, infection may be accompanied by a temperature elevation, leukocytosis, and a purulent discharge that is a product of dying leukocytes. Hypoxemia may be present in a person recoving from surgery with or without wound infection. By itself, hypoxemia is not a sign of infection. Mrs. P's hypoxemia may be related to hypoventilation and inadequate lung expansion. Ultimately, this will adversely effect healing as oxygen is needed to support cellular proliferation in the wound bed.

4. **c** decrease the wound dead space that may occur with accumulation of blood and fluid

Rationale

A drain is placed in the wound bed at the time of surgery to keep wound dead space at a minimum during healing. If blood is allowed to accumulate in the wound and form a clot, this will serve as a mechanical barrier to oxygen diffusion across the wound. Also, the dead cells that make up the clot will have to be cleared from the wound before normal healing can take place. Dead blood cells also provide an excellent culture medium for Escherichia coli bacteria, making it even more undesirable to have them present. Any blood in the wound can be readily evacuated through the drain. The drain also facilitates the removal of other fluid accumulations in the wound and, thus, minimizes edema. A drain is not put in place in anticipation of an infection but rather to help prevent one.

5. **c** high-pressure pulsatile irrigations

Rationale

Debridement of necrotic tissue is necessary before laying down of new and viable cells in the wound bed. Current research indicates that high-pressure pulsatile irrigation with a solution such as normal saline is most effective in ridding the wound bed of bacteria and debris. A very simple way to accomplish this is by the use of a 60-ml irrigating tip syringe. Wet to dry dressings will be effective in absorbing and pulling debris off the wound bed, but they will also pull off any fragile newly formed granulation tissue. If the use of a dressing is preferred for debridement, it is more appropriate and humane to use a wet to damp type of dressing. The petrolatum gauze being used in the management of Mrs. P.'s wound has some debriding properties and keeps the incision line free of dry crust formation that impedes cell migration. Betadine solution is nephrotoxic when used in full strength. It is also very desiccating and may, therefore, inhibit the formation of healthy new cells. Hydrogen peroxide should never be used as a dressing medium. It may be used to cleanse an incision line (preferably one-half strength), but it should always be rinsed off with normal saline to prevent destruction of viable tissue.

6. **c** glucose

Rationale

The most important nutrients during the defensive phase of wound healing are oxygen, protein, and glucose. Glucose is essential as an energy source, but it must be available intracellularly. For this reason, careful monitoring of Mrs. P.'s blood glucose is important so that insulin may be administered as needed to facilitate movement of glucose into the cell. Vitamin C, calcium, and iron are needed in wound healing mainly as cofactors for various biochemical reactions. Because only a minute amount of these nutrients is required in the cofactor role, there is seldom a problem with clinically significant deficiencies.

3 Acquired Immune Deficiency Syndrome (AIDS)

1. **c**   impaired functioning of one or more components of the immune/inflammatory response

   ### Rationale
   The HIV virus selects target cells (primarily CD4-positive T cells) to invade; there is evidence, however, that the virus also invades macrophages and nerve cells. The functioning of the B cell is also impaired, because of T-cell malfunction.

2. **b**   The HIV virus infects and kills the host T_4 cells, decreasing their numbers

   ### Rationale
   Because of its unique capabilities, the HIV virus infects and destroys T_4 cells, thereby depleting their numbers. As the number of T_4 cells decreases, the ratio declines. This is a major immunological finding in AIDS sufferers.

3. **d**   HIV is variable and often has a prolonged period of dormancy

   ### Rationale
   Like influenza, HIV has many genetic variants. The virus can remain dormant for many years so it would be difficult to demonstrate the efficacy of a vaccine.

4. **c**   the filling of the alveoli with eosinophilic exudate and PCP

   ### Rationale
   The alveoli filled with eosinophilic exudate and PCP, resulting in diminished to poor gas exchange. Pleural effusion, if present, is usually caused by Kaposi's sarcoma. D.L.'s nonproductive cough suggests that a bacterial respiratory infection is not present.

5. **a** reactivation of previously present microorganisms

   Rationale
   The majority of people have been infected with numerous microorganisms by the age of 4. These microorganisms are not pathogenic in immune competent individuals but cause severe diarrhea in immune compromised individuals. Common microorganisms include MAI, CMV, Cryptosporidium, and Histoplasma.

6. **d** presence of HIV virus in peripheral nerves and the central nervous system

   Rationale
   HIV virus targets neurological cells in the central nervous system and peripheral nerves, as well as T cells, probably through the macrophage. Toxoplasmosis tends to result in focal symptoms, such as seizures.

7. **b** cognitive, motor, and behavioral changes

   Rationale
   These three changes are present to a greater or lesser degree in the majority of individuals with AIDS.

8. **c** inability to eradicate infections associated with advanced stages of AIDS

   Rationale
   These ever-present microorganisms demonstrate a temporary response to medications but usually flare up as the medication is discontinued. Some therapies must be continued for the life of the individual.

4 Breast Cancer

1. **a** history of breast cancer in family members

   Rationale
   Cancer of the breast has been linked to a number of different risk factors. To date, however, only radiation has been demonstrated to cause damage to the deoxyribonucleic acid (DNA) structure that produces cellular mutations. A positive familial history of breast cancer (genetic predisposition) is the only risk factor that has consistently shown a strong positive causal link in research studies. Other factors that have been causally associated with breast cancer to varying degrees are an early onset of menarche and/or a late onset of menopause, nulliparity, mother's age at birth of first child, a past history of proliferative breast disease, ethnic background, and dietary patterns. With the exception of radiation exposure, researchers have no definitive answer for how these risk factors affect the incidence of breast cancer in the population. This lack of understanding is compounded by the fact that cancer is not one disease but many, with the potential for a variety of different causes.

2. **d** The lymph node is the result of cancer cells' spreading to different tissues within the body

   Rationale
   A devastating characteristic of cancer cells is their ability to spread (metastasize) to surrounding tissue structures. Cancer cells are frequently transported to the axillary nodes through the rich lymphatic channels that surround the breast. Approximately 75% of all breast cancers arise from the ductal epithelium and infiltrate the lymphatic drainage system. The portal of entry into the lymphatic system depends on the location of the breast tumor. A positive finding of axillary nodes on examination plays a key part in the clinical staging of breast cancer. If nodes are present, then there is the clinical indication that the cancer has spread from the primary site to another site in the body. This finding not only impacts treatment decisions but also affects the morbidity and mortality of the individual. The survival rate for individuals wtih breast cancer is much better for those diagnosed early in the course of the disease process. Early discovery has been demonstrated to increase survival rates and 5-year disease-free rates.

3. **b** The mass in the right breast is the result of a different pattern of cellular proliferation than that taking place in the left

Rationale

The cardinal characteristic of breast cancer tumors is a hard fixed mass that can adhere easily to either the nipple or the adjacent skin. Cancer cells have the ability to divide and multiply rapidly as well as infiltrate the surrounding areas in the search for essential nutrients. The clinical signs differ with the type of cells causing the occurrence. There are a number of different types of neoplastic cells that can arise from mammary epithelium. These cells can be either benign or malignant. Benign tumors result from cells that tend to mirror healthy cells more closely. Malignant tumors are the result of much more deviant cells, which are often anaplastic in nature. Malignant cells can be very different in structure and function from healthy cells.

4. **d** The remaining lymph nodes are inadequate to handle the lymph flow creating an increase in the hydrostatic pressure

Rationale

The lymphatic system fulfills three primary functions. It is part of the immune system and produces antibodies to fight foreign antigens. Although the swelling Mrs. C. is experiencing could be the result of an infectious process, her dressing has been dry and her temperature has not been elevated. The most probable cause of this symptom is the removal of lymph glands, which compromises the lymphatic flow, which creates a buildup of lymph drainage and leakage of this drainage into the interstitial spaces, creating lymphedema.

5. **d** All of the above

Rationale

Staging and classification of tumors have become important for physicians as both diagnostic and treatment tools. Staging has allowed researchers to examine how best to treat different categories of tumors as well as to have some sense of prognostic outcomes. Much of the standardized treatment regimens is based on the correlates of staging and treatment outcomes.

6. **a** Lymphedema can be aggravated by any kind of trauma to the hand from a cut, a burn, or anything causing prolonged pressure to the area

Rationale

Lymphedema can occur secondary to surgery shortly afterward, several weeks later, or months later. It is important for those who have had a mastectomy to understand this phenomenon. Individuals need to maintain the integrity of the first line of defense against infection. Any trauma that leads to a portal of entry for bacteria has the potential to cause infection and activate the body's immune response, resulting in lymphedema.

7. **d** Hormones will bind with the DNA in the nucleus, causing a transcription in the coding that affects cell viability

Rationale

Mrs. C.'s tumor was estrogen-sensitive, meaning that the tumor cells will respond to hormones. It is thought that hormones combine with the DNA in the nucleus of a cell and alter the ribonucleic acid (RNA) transcription process. This alteration is carried by the messenger RNA (mRNA), which controls the protein synthesis function of the cell. The biochemical disruption will interfere with cell viability.

1. **c**   Metastatic involvement

   Rationale
   Lung cancers frequently present initially with metastatic symptoms. His fixed and nontender nodes, neurological symptoms, and vague pain in arm and shoulder indicate metastatic involvement. Lung cancers are frequently diagnosed after metastatic involvement. This is usually due to the insidious onset of the disease in long-term smokers who are accustomed to respiratory problems and do not readily notice an increase or alteration in their respiratory status. The most common sites of metastatic lung cancer are the brain and bones, causing symptoms the individual cannot easily ignore.

2. **d**   all of the above

   Rationale
   Asbestos workers who smoke have an eightfold greater risk of lung cancers than individuals who work with asbestos and do not smoke. They have 92 times the risk of developing lung cancers of people who do not smoke and are not exposed to asbestos. In addition, living near a highway and a history of lung disease predispose Mr. G. to developing lung cancer.

3. **c**   He might suffer respiratory arrest

   Rationale
   Mr. G. has a history of symptoms associated with chronic obstructive pulmonary disease (COPD). Placing these individuals on oxygen satiates their chemoreceptors and may result in severe respiratory depression.

4. **a**   destruction of alveoli secondary to abuse (smoking) and disease

   Rationale
   Chronic long-term smoking results in breakdown of the fragile alveolar walls in the lungs. This results in less functional gas exchange as a result of the decrease in alveolar surface area. Over many years, this condition leads to clubbing of the fingers caused by inadequate oxygenation of the nailbeds, and in increased A-P chest diameter (barrel chest) secondary to an increased costovertebral angle. Additionally, Mr. G.'s other respiratory assessment findings are consistent with COPD and lung cancer. Findings include increased tactile fremitus, as sound waves travel better through a consolidated (solid) area than through an air-filled area, and dullness to percussion of this area secondary to a mass of tumor.

5. **d**   a tumor pressing on the bronchi or unilaterally, inhibiting air from entering the lower lobe without turbulence

   Rationale
   Wheezing is caused by turbulent air traveling at high speeds through a narrowed channel. Mr. G.'s wheeze is unilateral and on the right, where the area of consolidation (dullness to percussion and increased tactile fremitus) was located. This would indicate that the tumor mass is pressing upon the bronchi on the right, inhibiting free passage of air.

6. **d**   All of the above

   Rationale
   Cancer therapy in general revolves around destructon of tumor cells. As tumor cells multiply at roughly 25 times the rate of normal cells, their DNA and RNA synthesis is particularly vulnerable to effects of agents or therapies that inhibit this synthesis. Unfortunately, chemotherapy and radiation therapy are not exclusive in their destruction of cells. Healthy bone marrow, hair follicles, and gastrointestinal mucosa are destroyed in the process, causing alopecia, thrombocytopenia, and gastrointestinal disturbances. Anorexia, nausea, vomiting, and diarrhea are common side effects of chemotherapy as it is a systemic therapy. Radiation therapy affects those areas within the beam of radiation. In Mr. G.'s case, some esophagus tissue would likely be irritated in his lung fields. Irradiation of bone metastases would result in bone marrow depression within those bones, contributing to thrombocytopenia and pancytopenia.

6 Senile Dementia of the Alzheimer Type (SDAT)

1. **c** mental status examination and progressive course of the dementia

   Rationale

   A history of progressive cognitive deterioration over time and deficits in recent memory, concentration, and judgment (as measured on a mental status examination) are clinical indicators of SDAT and serve as the basis for diagnosis. There are also data that support a higher incidence of SDAT in individuals with a positive familial history of the disease. The differential diagnosis of dementia is often made by the exclusion of other disorders. The complete blood count and chemistry evaluations are important for ruling out various anemias and metabolic disorders that may be reversible causes of dementia. Mrs. K. may have an electrolyte imbalance caused by the use of a diuretic to manage her hypertension. The CT scan and electroencephalogram can also be used to identify other organic causes of dementia; however, evidence of changes in the brain tissue and its impulse conduction are often not evident in the early stages of SDAT. Past medical history, functional ability, and physical examination do not provide any disease specific markers.

2. **a** Depressed clients often complain of memory problems, whereas demented clients try to conceal memory impairment

   Rationale

   Demented persons characteristically hide and even confabulate to mask their problems with memory in the early stages of the disease. Depressed persons often state that they are having problems with their memory. Depression is marked by a rapid, often very time-specific onset. Depressed persons generally have a stable, apathetic, withdrawn pattern of behavior and poor self-image. In contrast, demented persons have an ill-defined onset of symptoms; dementia is marked by unpredictable fluctuating patterns of behavior. Demented persons also maintain a stable, unchanged self-image.

3. **b**   hypertension and cardiovascular diseases

Rationale

About 25% of demented persons have MID. Multiple brain infarctions are generally caused by thrombosis, hemorrhage, or emboli. The brain damage is permanent; however, if the underlying cardiovascular disease (i.e., hypertension) is treated, further brain infarctions can be prevented. Mrs. K. has a history of hypertension so she is at risk for MID. In the early stages, both MID and SDAT may exhibit essentially normal CT scan results. Later in the disease process, individuals have characteristic changes on their CT scans. MID clients have multiple lacunar infarcts or "holes" in their brain tissue, whereas SDAT presents with enlarged ventricles and widened sulci. It is also important to remember that MID and SDAT can coexist in one person.

4. **d**   It is used in small doses to control disruptive and destructive behavior

Rationale

Currently, available drug therapy for dementia is primarily for symptomatic relief and does not slow or reverse the course of the disease. Drugs that contain precursors to acetylcholine and others that stimulate brain metabolism are in clinical trials to document their impact on dementia. Major tranquilizers are not the drugs of choice for the treatment of depression.

Small doses of thioridazine, haloperidol, and thiothixene (all major tranquilizers) can be very useful in decreasing problematic behaviors in demented clients. Individuals can also have an "orienting" effect from these drugs. Side effects of these drugs must be weighed against benefits to the client. Side effects include drowsiness, further impairment of thought processes, and hypotension, increasing the person's risk for falling. Tardrive dyskinesia is a permanent disabling side effect. Control of eating, swallowing, and purposeful activities are decreased to rhythmic, repetitious motor movements.

5. **c**   pneumonia

Rationale

The person with SDAT becomes at risk for complications related to immobility. Lying in bed or sitting in chairs for long periods and bowel and bladder incontinence increase the incidence of skin breakdown. Healing is compromised because of poor nutrient intake. Dehydration from poor fluid intake increases the risk of urinary tract infections, incontinence, and poor perfusion of the kidneys. Death is most commonly caused by pneumonia.

6. **a**   neurofibrillary tangles and amyloid plaques

Rationale
The diagnosis of SDAT is made by pathological examination revealing the classic "tangles and plaques" in place of normal nerve cells in the brain. Cerebral atrophy is nonspecific but is a finding consistent with degenerative dementias.

Spinal Cord Injury

1. **b**   spinal shock

   Rationale
   After injury to the spinal cord, a sudden neurovascular shutdown, called *spinal shock*, is common. This may account for the decreased blood pressure and temperature and flaccid paralysis. Spinal shock can last from minutes to days to several weeks.

2. **c**   These findings are consistent with the C5 and C6 level injury

   Rationale
   Initial neurological examination demonstrated findings consistent with an intact spinal cord above C5. An injury at the level of C5 and C6 results in incomplete quadriplegia. His ability to demonstrate gross bicep movement but lack of intact triceps help to substantiate his diagnosis. Injury to the C5 and C6 spinal cord level interferes with nerve innervation to the biceps, triceps, and brachioradialis. A.D.'s fracture is common because this is the area of spine where maximum movement occurs.

3. **c**   He is breathing only with his diaphragm

   Rationale
   Respiratory failure is a danger in an individual with a spinal cord injury at the C5 and C6 level. The nerves that innervate the intercostal muscles are at this level. The diaphragmatic breathing remains intact and can be sufficient, but respiratory problems may arise because of the decreased vital capacity and ineffectiveness of his respirations.

4. **a**   He may develop a stress ulcer quickly

Rationale
Symptoms of stress ulcer will appear between the sixth and fourteenth days after injury. Any signs of anemia or blood in vomitus or stools must be reported immediately. Spinal cord shock triggers a physiological stress response that includes the inhibition of gastrointestinal activity and an increase in the release of stress hormones that affect gastric acidity. This condition may be complicated by the use of steroidal drugs to decrease spinal cord swelling. This condition is difficult to detect as a result of the paresthesia below the level of injury. Otherwise, the individual may report pain. A report of shoulder pain in the quadriplegic individual should be explored, as it may be referred pain from the abdomen.

5. **d**   rectal suppository followed by digital stimulation

Rationale
The rectum will respond to the suppository within several minutes by expelling it and the contents of the sigmoid colon. Eventually, after the bowel senses the suppository at the same time daily, all that will be necessary will be the digital stimulus to evacuate the bowel. If nothing happens initially, it may be necessary to remove stool in the lower bowel. Sufficient fluids, a diet adequate in roughage, and stool softeners and/or laxatives may help augment the situation. If there are no results within 3 to 5 days, an enema may be ordered to stimulate evacuation.

6. **b**   Intermittent catheterizations will help maintain bladder tone and prevent infections

Rationale
Reflex activity may return to the bladder because the nerves at the area of the sacrum that innervate the bladder may return after spinal shock. If intermittent catheterization is instituted, it will be important that fluid intake and elimination balance. Overdistension of the bladder may destroy the detrusor muscle's ability to contract, jeopardizing the return of autonomic function after spinal shock. The intervals between catheterizations, every 4 hours at first, may be adjusted according to the amount of urine obtained. After a pattern of elimination is established, spontaneous voiding may be elicited by stimulating the sacral reflex arc, using thigh stroking or Crede's method, depending on the injury at the upper or lower motor neuron. If spontaneous voiding does not occur, intermittent catheterization may continue.

7. **c**   He may indeed be able to have erections, but the necessary ejaculation may not occur for some time or may never occur

Rationale

Loss of sensation of the genitals occurs in complete cord injuries. Males with upper motor neuron injuries have reflexogenic erections, usually caused by cutaneous stimulation. Those with lower motor neuron injuries do not have the reflexogenic erection but may be able to have psychogenic erections by using erotic stimulations of sight, sound, smell, and touch. Although male fertility is usually reduced considerably as a result of the nervous system's lack of ability to coordinate ejaculation, many male quadriplegics have some form of sexual expression, although it may not be in the form of producing a child.

Cerebral Vascular Accident (CVA)

1. **b**   thrombosis with an ischemic event

   Rationale

   Mostly likely classified as a reversible ischemic neurological deficit (RIND) rather than a transient ischemic attack (TIA). A RIND lasts longer than 12 to 24 hours (symptoms can last days or weeks) with minimal, partial, or no deficit. A TIA lasts no longer than 24 hours with no residual dysfunction.

   A thrombus is a primary occlusion of a major cerebral vessel or a branch of the middle cerebral artery. Ms. R. has a history of atherosclerosis as evidenced by a previous femoral-popliteal bypass surgery. The decreased pressure in the ophthalmic artery indicates carotid lumen narrowing. The lumbar puncture was clear and colorless, and the opening pressure indicated no increased intracranial pressure, which frequently accompanies a cerebral hemorrhage. Blood in the cerebrospinal fluid is a positive sign for a subarachnoid hemorrhage. Embolic stroke was ruled out by a normal electrocardiogram. Atrial fibrillation or presence of heart disease would indicate the heart as a source of emboli. There was no evidence of deep vein thrombosis.

2. **f**   all of the above

   Rationale

   According to the National Center for Health Statistics, CVA ranked third as the cause of adult deaths. Investigators have found a direct relationship between increased blood vessel disease and the following risk factors: cigarette smoking, diabetes mellitus, hypertension, elevated cholesterol, obesity, sedentary life style, family history, and high-estrogen oral contraceptive use in women.

3. **d**   a, b

Rationale

When an artery becomes occluded, a decrease in the blood supply to that portion of the brain it supplies causes ischemia, resulting in cell death and hypoxia. Brain ischemia produces a loss of electrical activity affecting the sodium and potassium pump mechanism in the brain cells. In the absence of such pumping, increased sodium, followed by water, enters the cells, causing intracellular edema within 3 minutes. This edema causes increased swelling around the ischemic area, thus involving a larger portion of the brain than just the initial event.

4. **e**   checking the stool and urine for occult blood

Rationale

Bleeding from mucous membranes or any organ is always a potential hazard when an individual's clotting factors are disrupted by anticoagulants.

5. **d**   When a moderately sharp object strokes the lateral aspect of the sole from the heel to the ball of the foot, the response is dorsiflexion of the great toe and fanning of the small toes indicating upper motor neuron disease

Rationale

The motor system is divided into upper and lower motor neurons. Lower motor neurons are all neurons of the somatic, visceral, and brachial efferent cell columns which send motor axons into the peripheral nerves. Upper motor neurons send impulses from the cerebral cortex, or the brainstem, to activate lower motor neurons. No upper motor neuron axons leave the neuraxis. The pyramidal tract is the upper motor neuron pathway for voluntary movement.

Normal plantar response is flexion of the great toe to noxious stimuli. The most reliable sign of upper motor neuron or pyramidal tract disease is extension of the great toe in response to plantar stimulation. The reason for the change in flexion to extension of the great toe is unknown.

6. **c**   a narrowing of the carotid artery associated with atherosclerosis of the lumen

Rationale

Bruits and heart murmurs have identical physiological explanations. Both are caused by turbulent blood flow, though murmurs can have very different pathology. One of the most common causes of turbulent blood flow is the narrowing of a vessel. In Ms. R.'s case, the carotid artery has become narrowed as a result of atherosclerotic changes and the turbulent flow is heard as a bruit.

7. **c**   Restoration of normal perfusion pressure to the internal carotid system by surgery

Rationale

The digital angiogram indicated narrowing of both carotid arteries with evidence of ulcerated plaques

Ms. R. recovered from her surgery. The following behaviors are adopted: she stopped smoking; decreased weight to 125 pounds; walks 1 mile/day; follows a low-salt diet; and takes a diuretic to control blood pressure.

Bacterial Meningitis

1. **e**   all of the above

Rationale

Pneumococcal meningitis is most common in the very young and those over 40 years of age. It is also generally preceded by an infection located in some other place in the body. The most common sites for these infections are the respiratory tract, paranasal sinuses, oropharynx and nasopharynx, and ears. Under conditions that are not clearly understood, organisms from these sites can enter the blood stream and localize themselves in the meninges. The meninges have a particular affinity for the three bacteria that commonly cause meningitis (*Diplococcus pneumoniae, Haemophilus influenzae,* and *Neisseria meningitidis*). Individuals who are immunosuppressed for any reason are at even higher risk for transfer of infection. Causes of immunosuppression include chronic illness, immunosuppressive agents or antimetabolites, poor nutritional levels (frequently seen in alcoholics), defects in PMN leukocyte function, malignancy, and radiation therapy. It should also be noted that the central nervous system itself has a low resistance to infection; microorganisms of relatively low pathogenicity may cause an overwhelming infection when introduced to the central nervous system.

2. **d**   cerebrospinal fluid glucose of 30 mg/dl

Rationale

Although the cerebrospinal fluid pressure is elevated, it cannot be concluded that the pressure elevation is the result of infection. There are many causes of increased intracranial pressure and thus elevated cerebrospinal fluid pressure. The few red blood cells that are present are probably produced by the trauma of the lumbar puncture itself. The markedly elevated level of white blood cells in the blood is consistent with a bacterial infection, but not necessarily restricted to the central nervous system: pneumonia could have caused the elevation. A cerebrospinal fluid glucose level less than 40% of the serum glucose is almost always an indication of an infectious central nervous system process. The bacteria quickly consume the glucose that is present in the cerebrospinal fluid, making it a very good culture medium. There are other laboratory findings that, in conjunction with the low glucose, suggest meningitis in this case. The cerebrospinal fluid examination demonstrated an elevation of protein and the presence of a large number of white blood cells. The fact that the cells were predominantly PMNs is very suggestive of a bacterial process. The most significant finding was the presence of gram-positive diplococci in the cerebrospinal fluid.

3. **c**   some disorder of the cortical neurons, whose exact etiology is unknown

Rationale

Consciousness is an organism's awareness of its environment and its ability to react to internal and external stimuli. The two components of consciousness are content and level. Examples of content of consciousness are speech, orientation, rational thought, and judgment. *Level of consciousness* refers to a measure on a continuum between fully awake and totally unresponsive to any stimuli. Having a normal consciousness implies that the cerebral hemispheres and the reticular activating system within the brain stem are intact and functional. When a portion of the cerebral hemispheres is interrupted, specific content of consciousness will be disturbed (aphasia and disorientation are only two examples of many). When the damage to the cerebral hemispheres is extensive enough, or a more specific lesion interrupts the reticular activating system, the individual's level of consciousness is affected.

In the early stage of Mr. C.'s course, he became disoriented and confused. This interruption of the content of consciousness was probably caused by interruption of the normal function of the neurons within the central nervous system, specifically the cerebral cortex. Even though meningitis predominantly affects the meninges, specifically the pia and arachnoid layers, there is nearly always some degree of cerebritis (the exact cause is unknown). It may result from diffusion of toxins from the meninges, or circulatory disturbances, or some other factor. It is known, however, that the first effect of bacteria on the meninges is to cause hyperemia of the meningeal vessels. Shortly thereafter there occurs a migration of neutrophils into the subarachnoid space. The subarachnoid exudate increases, particularly over the base of the brain, and extends into the sheaths of the cranial and spinal nerves and, for a short distance, into the perivascular spaces of the cortex. It should be noted, however, that the changes that result in alteration of consciousness are not caused by the presence of bacteria in the substance of the brain and should, therefore, not be regarded as infectious encephalopathy. At this stage, it is unlikely that the alteration of consciousness is due to decreased generalized cerebral perfusion or herniation syndrome that might result from increased intracranial pressure.

4. **b** The blood-brain barrier limits entry of the antibiotic into the cerebrospinal fluid

Rationale

The blood-brain barrier has been described as a network of cells and membranes that are in close approximation with the capillary walls and the neurons. These include the epithelial cells of the capillary walls and the processes of glial astrocyte cells. The relationship between the capillary wall and the glial cell is the blood-brain barrier. The blood-cerebrospinal fluid barriers provide separations that are very selective in terms of membrane permeability. Most drugs are prevented from affecting the brain and spinal cord, but some are allowed to pass through the barrier. The movement of substances into the brain depends on particle size, lipid solubility, chemical dissociation, and protein-binding potential of the drug. In general, drugs that are lipid-soluble and undissociated at body pH rapidly enter the brain and cerebrospinal fluid. Water-soluble molecules and ions do not pass the barrier.

Chloramphenicol is a commonly used drug for central nervous system infections because of its propensity to pass easily into the cerebrospinal fluid. Cerebrospinal fluid concentration of Chloramphenicol is 30% to 80% of plasma concentration. In general, *Pneumococcus* is very sensitive to chloramphenicol as it is to penicillin. Penicillin, however, does not cross the barrier well. In fact, the only time that penicillin is able to cross the barrier is during infectious processes such as meningitis, when the barrier is disrupted. At that time, cerebrospinal fluid concentrations may reach 10% to 30% of the serum level. Newer drugs, that pass easily into the cerebrospinal fluid, including "new-generation" cephalosporins, are being developed now.

5. **d** hydrocephalus and cerebral edema

Rationale

As the infectious process continues, more and more fibrinopurulent exudate accumulates in the subarachnoid space. Hydrocephalus is produced by exudate in Magendie's foramen and Luschka's foramina, or in the subarachnoid space around the pons and the midbrain, interfering with the flow or reabsorption of cerebrospinal fluid. Later, fibrous subarachnoid adhesions may create additional interruption of cerebrospinal fluid circulation, compounding the problem further. This latter problem may result in chronic hydrocephalus. The results of hydrocephalus are twofold. First, it produces increased intracranial pressure to the extent that cerebral perfusion is decreased. This causes generalized decreased metabolic function of the brain that results in a decreased level of consciousness. Second, hydrocephalus may result in a herniation syndrome in which direct pressure is applied by supratentorial structures on the brain stem. This also causes a decreased level of consciousness. The mild amount of cerebral edema that results from the cerebritis only increases the intracranial pressure and contributes to all of the above.

6. **a** to remove intracellular and extracellular fluid from the brain

Rationale
Osmotic (hyperosmolar) diuretic agents are used primarily to remove fluid from the brain. Osmotic diuretics act by creating an osmotic gradient across the blood-brain barrier. This gradient draws intracellular and extracellular fluid from the brain into the intravascular space. In addition to their specific effect on the brain, these agents create an osmotic gradient between the blood and all tissues of the body. This leads to a greatly increased intravascular volume that perfuses the kidney. Marked diuresis follows the administration of these agents. The relative dehydration created within the brain results in a reduction of brain "volume". In addition to the direct reduction of intracranial volume, the marked diuresis also reduces the overall circulating blood volume, thus reducing the cerebral blood flow and therefore further reducing intracranial volume and pressure. These agents are used when immediate intervention is essential. This often gives the body an opportunity to mobilize its own compensatory mechanisms.

Hyperthyroidism: Graves
Disease

1. **d**   autoimmune response

   Rationale
   Although thyroid carcinoma and pituitary tumors can cause hyperthyroidism,
   they do not cause Graves disease. Hyperplasia is a result of, rather than a cause
   of, hyperthyroidism. The cause of Graves disease is thought to be an autoimmune response. In autoimmune conditions, the body produces antibodies that
   act against its own organs and tissues. Certain immunoglobulins, called thyroid-stimulating immunoglobulins (TSIs), are found in 95% of persons with
   Graves disease and are thought to be evidence of this autoimmune process. The
   TSIs are believed to bind themselves to thyroid-stimulating hormone (TSH)
   receptor sites in the thyroid cells, leading to increased activity of the thyroid
   gland.

2. **a**   negative feedback loop involving the anterior pituitary, thyroid, and hypothalamus

   Rationale
   In order to understand hyperthyroidism, one must first understand the normal
   production and regulation of thyroid hormones. In response to a fall in circulating thyroid hormones, the hypothalamus produces a substance called thy-
   rotropin-releasing hormone (TRH). TRH enters the blood stream and is carried
   to the anterior pituitary gland. In response to TRH, the anterior pituitary produces thyroid-stimulating hormone (TSH). When TSH is released, it binds with
   specific receptor sites on the membranes of thyroid cells. Once bound to receptors, TSH activates the thyroid gland to release its stored hormones and to produce more. Triiodothyronine (T_3) and thyroxine (T_4) are the thyroid hormones
   released into the blood stream. It is thought that T_3 is the active form of the
   hormone and has the greater action on the target organs. Normally, the
   increased levels of thyroid hormone act to inhibit the production of TRH and
   TSH. This is a *negative feedback loop*, so named because the thyroid hormones
   have a negative or inhibiting effect on TRH and TSH.

In Graves disease, the mechanisms that regulate thyroid hormone production are overridden. The thyroid gland secretes an abnormally high amount of thyroid hormone, which in turn suppresses TRH and TSH. Since the normal negative feedback loop is not operational, reduced TSH does not decrease the amount of thyroid hormone being released. T_3 and T_4 levels are, thus, increased, as is the body's uptake of iodine.

3. **c**   exophthalmos

Rationale
There are two types of eye problems that may occur with Graves disease. First, globe and lid lag may occur with certain eye movements. These are caused by the overactivity of the sympathetic nervous system in hyperthyroidism and usually resolve with treatment. Second, exophthalmos (proptosis, bulging eyes) is an example of an ophthalmopathy that does not resolve with treatment of hyperthyroidism. The eyes bulge because of edema (increased fluid) of the orbital contents. Other changes that may be seen with exophthalmos include paralysis of the eye muscles and retinal/optic nerve damage. It is thought that these changes are the result of an autoimmune antigen-antibody reaction that is distinct from the one leading to hyperthyroidism.

The individual may experience blurred or double vision from the muscle paralysis, decreased visual fields, photophobia, ocular pain, increased tearing, and corneal ulceration. Reversal of the hyperthyroidism does not cure these eye problems, though they may stabilize after treatment.

4. **d**   none of the above

Rationale
Goiter is an enlargement of the thyroid gland and commonly occurs with either hypothyroidism or hyperthyroidism. As such, it represents a compensatory mechanism triggered by altered thyroid hormone output. The thyroid gland hypertrophies (the cells increase in size) and becomes hyperplastic (the number of cells increases). Though it seems contradictory that the thyroid increases in size in both hypo- and hyperthyroid states, it makes sense when one remembers that the body is attempting to produce more thyroid hormone in both instances, though the pathologic mechanisms are nearly opposite.

Another type of goiter, called *nontoxic nodular goider*, can also be found in euthyroid states. The initial impetus for increasing the size of the thyroid gland arises from an increased demand for thyroid hormones, for example, from pregnancy or iodine deficiency. Though the gland usually returns to normal size when the need for more thyroid hormone resolves, it remains enlarged in some cases. However, changes in the thyroid cells allow the body to maintain normal levels of thyroid hormone, despite the enlarged gland. This results in a euthyroid, or balanced, state.

5. **b** increased basal metabolic rate, increased oxygen consumption, sympathetic stimulation

Rationale

One of the major functions of thyroid hormone is to regulate the body's basal metabolic rate; the rate at which the body metabolizes nutrients into energy and its by-products. In hyperthyroidism, the increased thyroid hormone causes an increase in the metabolic rate, often as much as 60% to 100%. The rate at which the body uses fats, carbohydrates, and protein speeds up, decreasing circulating cholesterol levels. A more pronounced effect is weight loss caused by the increased use of calories by the body. Individuals with hyperthyroidism may need 4000 to 5000 calories per day to maintain their weight. In addition, one of the end products of metabolism is heat; thus, in hyperthyroidism, the body produces unusually large amounts of heat. Blood flow to the skin increases in an effort to rid the body of this excess heat, leading to vasodilation and perspiration.

When metabolism increases, the body's oxygen consumption also increases, since oxygen is an integral part of metabolism. The body responds by increasing heart rate and cardiac output to provide the needed oxygen to the tissues. There is thought to be an interaction between the thyroid hormone and the sympathetic nervous system. Thyroid hormone either directly stimulates the sympathetic nervous system or makes the body more sensitive to catecholamines. In either case, tachycardia, heart palpitations, sweating, anxiety, and diarrhea may result from increased sympathetic activity. Therefore, the combination of increased metabolism, increased oxygen consumption, and increased sympathetic activity account for most of Ms. R.'s symptoms.

6. **b** destroys thyroid tissue and stops production of thyroid hormone

Rationale

The treatment of hyperthyroidism can be medical or surgical. Certain drugs, such as propylthiouracil and methimazole, are given to decrease production of thyroid hormone or to block its actions. Other drugs, such as propranolol, are given to decrease the sympathetic response to thyroid hormone. These are not usually considered to produce permanent control of hyperthyroidism and would probably not be viable options for hyperthyroidism as severe as Ms. R.'s.

Oral radioactive iodine is a nonsurgical, permanent treatment for hyperthyroidism. On entering the blood stream, it becomes concentrated in the thyroid cells and destroys them. This naturally destroys the body's ability to produce thyroid hormone. Surgical removal of the thyroid is another permanent solution to hyperthyroidism. After either of these treatments, Ms. R. would have to use exogenous thyroid for the rest of her life to meet her body's need for the hormone.

1. **b** white race

   Rationale
   To date, epidemiological studies suggest that type I diabetes mellitus is 1 1/2 to 2 times more common in whites than in nonwhites. The reason for this is unknown, and the incidence is often reversed in type II diabetes mellitus. The fact that S.S. is female has little or no relation to her developing diabetes mellitus. Type I diabetes mellitus is actually more common in males, although it affects females at an earlier age. No association with familial endocrine diseases, such as hypothyroidism, has been shown. S.S.'s risk of developing type I diabetes mellitus actually decreases with increasing age. The peak incidence of type I diabetes mellitus is 11 to 13 years. The risk of developing type II diabetes mellitus, however, increases with age.

2. **b** lack of functioning insulin

   Rationale
   In type I diabetes mellitus, no functional insulin is produced. Although a variety of theories exist to explain the etiology of type I diabetes mellitus, it should never be confused with non-insulin-dependent diabetes mellitus (type II DM). Many experts consider the two types of diabetes mellitus to represent two entirely different diseases. However, considerable evidence does suggest that type I diabetes mellitus is characterized by both a lack of insulin and a relative excess in glycagon. In this case history, the lack of insulin caused an accumulation of glucose in the blood. As S.S.'s renal threshold was exceeded, the glucose spilled into the urine. The large glucose molecules acted as an osmotic diuretic, resulting in the loss of much water in the urine. Thus, S.S. voided large amounts at frequent intervals. Similarly, although she ate large amounts of food, weight loss occurred because of both the fluid loss and body tissue depletion as fats and proteins were used for energy.

3. **c**   before cheerleading practice

Rationale

Insulin will be needed in greatest quantity postprandially (after meals) in order to normalize blood glucose levels effectively and stimulate fatty acid and amino acid uptake by cells. Hormones that are released during times of stress, such as emotional stress or during an illness or injury actually antagonize insulin, and many produce an increased need of insulin. Exercise, however, may precipitate severe hypoglycemia when performed after the administration of insulin. Thus, insulin requirements are diminished with exercise.

Cheerleading practice involves a great deal of exercise. S.S. should appropriately decrease the rate of insulin injection before practice. She may also need to increase her food intake before practice.

4. **b**   sufficient in calories to maintain normal weight

Rationale

Although excessive intake of calories is detrimental to all individuals with diabetes mellitus, it is important that S.S.'s caloric and nutrient intake be sufficient for normal growth and development. She is an active girl who is still growing. In addition, she is thin and has lost several pounds. She should consume adequate amounts of carbohydrates, fats, and proteins in a well-balanced diet. Most of the fats should be unsaturated to decrease the incidence of vascular changes. The carbohydrates should be complex rather than simple to provide a more constant blood glucose level. Food intake should be congruent with cultural, social, and ethnic circumstances. There is no reason for her to miss socializing with her friends over food, providing she consumes proper kinds of food. Pizza, hamburgers, and other "fast foods" may be consumed on the American Diabetic Association (ADA) diet.

5. **a**   neurological malnutrition

Rationale

S.S. has experienced an episode of hypoglycemia caused by an accidental overdose of insulin. Symptoms of hypoglycemia may result from adrenergic reaction or cellular malnutrition. However, the symptoms experienced by S.S. are occurring because her neurons are receiving inadequate supplies of metabolizable carbohydrates to maintain their normal function. Other symptoms would predominate in both diabetic ketoacidosis (DKA) and hypersomolar hyperglycemic nonketotic coma (HHNK). She should immediately ingest a source of glucose, such as orange juice or hard candy.

6. **d** has an absolute deficiency of insulin with an increase in stress hormones

Rationale
S.S. has developed DKA because she has no insulin and is encountering a stressful situation in the form of flu. Although she is not eating, her body continues to form glucose. By discontinuing her insulin, she allows her serum glucose level to rise. The rising glucose causes a solute diuresis, much like the one she experienced when first diagnosed with diabetes mellitus. This alerts her to the fact that there is a problem. In addition, however, the decreased insulin level results in excessive ketone formation. The ketones are not efficiently used by the tissues and thus accumulate in the body. When S.S. tested her urine, she found it positive for acetone. Acetone is less toxic than the ketones ß-hydroxybutyrate and acetoacetic acids but is more easily measured. Although a growth spurt and lack of food intake could contribute to metabolic problems, her DKA has occurred primarily because of her insulin deficiency and stress hormone level increase. She should never discontinue her insulin for any significant period of time.

7. **a** microvascular disease

Rationale
Microvascular disease, particularly involving the retina and kidneys, is often the earliest common sequela for individuals with type I diabetes mellitus. The frequency of microvascular disease correlates with the duration of the disease. Thickening of the basement membrane of the capillaries occurs slowly. Retinal and renal changes result. Although macrovascular disease does occur in type I diabetes mellitus, the manifestations of coronary artery disease and cerebral vascular accident occur much later than microvascular manifestations. Sexual disorders may occur but will not ordinarily occur early in the course of diabetes mellitus. Other endocrine dysfunction may occur at any time.

8. **c** proteinuria

Rationale
The first, most typical manifestation of renal dysfunction in individuals with type I diabetes mellitus is proteinuria. The exact mechanism responsible for the increased permeability of capillaries is unknown. However, the leakage of albumin into glomerular filtrate results in albuminuria. Proteinuria is usually noted routinely after 10 to 15 years of insulin treatment. S.S. has been treated with insulin for 12 years. Urinary protein losses may reach 10 to 30 g daily, resulting in hypoproteinemia. Because of the reduction in plasma osmotic pressure, severe generalized edema (anasarca) and hypertension may occur. As renal function deteriorates, both the serum creatine and the blood urea nitrogen levels increase. The development of Kimmelstiel-Wilson nodules does occur in individuals with type I diabetes mellitus but does not necessarily precede the proteinuria. The nodules may not be noted until a diagnostic test, such as intravenous pyelogram (IVP), is conducted or until kidney biopsy results are known.

1. **b** excessive levels of circulating cortisol

   Rationale
   Mrs. S.'s clinical signs and symptoms are caused by hypercortisolism. Circulating ACTH and cortisol levels are normally controlled by negative feedback. As ACTH increases, there is an increase in cortisol, which in turn decreases ACTH production. In Mrs. S.'s case, the anterior pituitary is constantly producing excessive ACTH, which does not respond to the increased cortisol levels. As a result, ACTH increases the levels of both cortisol and adrenal androgens. Administration of pharmaceutical cortisone preparations, especially in high doses, can precipitate symptoms.

2. **d** urinary cortisol decrease with high levels of dexamethasone

   Rationale
   The dexamethasone suppression test helps to determine the underlying cause of Mrs. S.'s symptoms. The pathophysiology of Cushing's syndrome relates to pituitary-dependent hypercortisolism. High doses of dexamethasone are necessary to produce a mild effect on ACTH produced by the anterior pituitary. One would normally expect a significant drop in cortisol levels as dexamethasone effectively suppresses normal levels of ACTH secretion. When hypercortisolism is caused by an adrenal tumor, no change will be seen. At the present time, Mrs. S.'s laboratory values show that her cortisol is adequately suppressing high ACTH levels but she is experiencing complications resulting from the high intake of cortisol. Blood tests to be taken 1 month from now will help determine the cortisol dosage that will still be effective in lowering the ACTH levels while diminishing some current side effects.

3. **c**   protein wasting and collagen loss

Rationale

As a result of long-term cortisol therapy, increased protein breakdown (catabolism) leads to loss of adipose and lymphatic tissue. Protein wasting can result in collagen loss, causing individuals to bruise easily. Loss of the collagenous support around vessels makes them susceptible to rupture from insignificant events. Lack of collagen also leads to thin, atrophic skin.

4. **d**   A diet restricted in sodium and complex carbohydrates is needed

Rationale

Taking cortisone results in changes in carbohydrate, lipid, and protein metabolism. Alterations include increases in gluconeogenesis, blood glucose, and protein catabolism. Cortisone also increases appetite. With these alterations in metabolism, weight gain is a common problem. Overt diabetes mellitus results from these metabolic changes in some individuals.

Mrs. S. needs dietary counseling as she is at risk for diabetes mellitus and atherosclerosis because of the pathological metabolic alterations. A low-calorie diet, following the recommendations of the American Diabetic Association and the American Heart Association, would be the diet of choice. In addition, regular exercise is recommended as a weight-reducing measure. Regular exercise, involving the muscles that Mrs. S. feels are weakest, will help increase their strength. Exercise is also an excellent method of enhancing well-being and, indirectly, treating depression.

5. **3**   b, c, d

Rationale

The major causes of death in those with Cushing's syndrome are related to untreated infections, hypertensive disease, depression, and arteriosclerosis. It is important to monitor blood pressure for signs of hypertension. Mrs. S. also needs to avoid illness and infection because of increased susceptibility. In addition, her physiologic stress response has been altered.

1. **c , d** Hemolytic anemia and B_{12} deficiency (pernicious)

   ### Rationale

   Iron deficiency is one likely initial choice of diagnosis. Anemia of chronic disease also results in microcytic, hypochromic red cells with decreased levels of hemoglobin and hematocrit, but her history indicates that she has been healthy and has not experienced chronic illness. Pernicious anemia and hemolytic anemias tend to produce macrocytic red cells. She is of Greek heritage, which increases the likelihood of the thalassemias as etiology of her anemia; both produce hypochromic, microcytic erythrocytes.

2. **a** decreased serum ferritin, increased TIBC, increased FEP

   ### Rationale

   Serum ferritin is one of the most sensitive tests for isolating iron deficiency anemia, along with TIBC and FEP increases. Folate, B_{12}, bilirubin, and reticulocyte counts are normal for both thalassemia and iron deficiency anemia. Serum iron and transferrin are both extremely labile laboratory measures and can vary diurnally in healthy individuals as much as 30% to 40%.

3. **c** shift to the right

   ### Rationale

   The curve would shift to the right. The body tries to compensate for the hypoxia it experiences secondary to anemia by shifting to the right, facilitating removal of more oxygen by the tissues while maintaining the same partial pressure of oxygen.

4. **b**   tachycardia

Rationale

The body tries to compensate for the anemia-induced hypoxia in several ways: (1) shift of the oxyhemoglobin dissociation curve to the right; (2) blood redistribution (shunting) away from tissues with abundant blood supply but low oxygen requirement (e.g., skin) to tissues with higher oxygen needs (e.g., brain, muscle, heart); (3) increased cardiac output through increased heart rate or stroke volume; and/or (4) increased rate of erythrocyte production in 4 to 5 days. Glossitis and cheilitis are frequently associated with the anemias. Tachypnea reflects decreased oxygen-carrying capacity of the erythrocytes. The newly developed cardiac murmur is commonly associated with anemia and results from an increase in quantity and speed of low-viscosity blood passing through the cardiac chambers.

5. **d**   blood loss

Rationale

Blood loss is the major cause of iron deficiency anemia among Americans. Ms. I.'s history reveals multiple factors that could contribute to anemia from blood loss.

1. A history of menorrhagia, possible exacerbated by her IUD. Menorrhagia is defined as blood loss of more than 60 ml/cycle. A "normal" woman may lose 17 to 30 mg of iron each menstrual period in addition to expected daily losses of around 1 mg through the skin, sweat, and urine.

2. Excessive use of aspirin each cycle. Aspirin is a gastric irritant that can precipitate microhemorrhage from the gastrointestinal tract.

3. Butazolidin, like other anti-inflammatory medications, is a gastrointestinal irritant with a potential for causing aplastic anemia.

4. Finally, methydopate hydrochloride (Aldomet) has been implicated as a potential cause of hemolytic anemia.

There are many other etiologies for the various anemias. These include (1) renal dysfunction with decreased erythropoietin production; (2) presence of prosthetic heart valves, causing erythrocyte hemolysis; (3) malabsorption (diabetic or other diarrhea, sprue, surgical resection of the small bowel); (4) medication-induced (carbamazepine [Tegretol], phenytoin sodium [Dilantin], intravenous infusion [Septra], steroids, anticoagulants); (5) frank blood loss (ulcers, hemorrhoids, trauma, ulcerative colitis); (6) possible maliganancy (should always be ruled out); (7) excessive blood donation (more than 3 times/year); and/or (8) dietary causes (anorexia, poverty). However, these may be associated with other types of anemia, as well as iron deficiency.

6. **c** ferrous sulfate 325 mg by mouth three times a day, given with orange juice

Rationale

Oral iron replacement is preferred to parenteral for the vast majority of individuals. Intramuscular injection is painful and can stain the skin. Z-tract technique should be used. Oral iron is best absorbed in an acid medium (i.e., either an empty duodenum or with orange juice). Ferrous fumerate actually contains the highest iron content of all available oral preparations (35% as compared to 20% iron in ferrous sulfate). However, when taken with antacids the iron salt is chelated, thus making it unavailable for absorption. Other drugs that may interfere with iron absorption include allopurinol (Zyloprim), cholestyramine resin (Questran), pancreatic enzyme extracts, and possibly vitamin E. A multicomponent hematinic is inappropriate; Ms. I. has normal levels of folate and B_{12}. Calcium in the mix will interfere with iron absorption. Ms. I.'s anemia is considered moderate (hemoglobin 6 to 10 g). Transfusion is considered a last resort and only for severe anemia with life-threatening symptoms.

7. **b** no

Rationale

Ms. I. might notice less nausea, but constipation and black tarry stools are expected side effects of iron therapy. Enteric coated and timed release preparations are not recommended because they transport the iron past the duodenum and proximal jejunum, where 90% of iron absorption occurs. She may need to decrease the dose of oral iron if these symptoms become too bothersome.

8. **d** green leafy vegetables, liver, citrus fruits

Rationale

Foods with little color are often poor sources of iron. Chicken, rice, potatoes, cereal, milk, eggs, and toast are low in iron. Iron is poorly absorbed from eggs, even though the yolk has a good supply. Milk, like antacids, inhibits iron absorption, as does the tannin in tea and phytase in many cereals. Citrus fruits and green vegetables also contain high quantities of vitamin C, which aids in iron absorption. It has been recommended that women of childbearing age ingest 18 mg of iron a day. Without special enrichment or exogenous supplements, a woman would have to take in at least 3000 calories daily to provide this quantity of iron.

9. c   hemoglobin and MCV

Rationale

Two thirds of a hemoglobin deficit will be corrected after 1 month of therapeutic iron regardless of the severity. Sources suggest that individuals continue iron for about 1 year after the source of the bleeding has been corrected. Hemoglobin and MCV are the most accurate tests to indicate improvement of iron and size of the red cell. Hematocrit will only indicate the volume percentage of erythrocytes. MCHC is very insensitive, being a mathematically derived value. Reticulocyte count was normal initially and no significant change is expected. Bone marrow aspiration is a painful, costly procedure that might be performed if routine blood tests did not reveal the exact nature of the hematologic defect. Since it was not necessary for her initial diagnosis, it certainly is not indicated for routine follow-up.

1. **c**   petechiae and unexplained ecchymosis

   Rationale
   The onset of ALL is usually insidious. Signs include general malaise, fatigue, anorexia, and history of recent viral infection from which the child appears not to have fully recovered. Fortunately, fatigue and anorexia are usually found to be symptoms of a less serious problem. Palpable, nontender lymph nodes are not an uncommon finding in young children because the lymphatic system comprises almost double the amount of tissue in children that it does in adults. The presence of petechiae or unexplained ecchymosis is always abnormal and must be further investigated with complete blood count, differential, and platelet count.

2. **d**   10% blasts

   Rationale
   Although the hemoglobin, total white count, and thrombocytes all have abnormal values, they could be explained by different causes (anemia, infection, and idiopathic thrombocytopenic purpura, respectively). The presence of blasts in the peripheral blood sample indicates a bone marrow dysfunction. The hallmark of acute leukemia is the presence of blast cells. Blast cells are a part of the normal maturation sequence of hemic and lymphoid elements, however, they constitute less than 5% of the nucleated cells of the bone marrow and are never found in the peripheral blood. With leukemia, the bone marrow changes from the production of mature, functional cells to abnormal, undifferentiated cells.

3. **b**   no

Rationale

There are only a few known high-risk factors for leukemia. The most striking is the incidence of leukemia in an identical twin of a child with leukemia. People who have received irradiation for polycythemia vera or ankylosing spondylitis and atomic bomb survivors are also at risk. The last group at risk for childhood leukemia are children with chromosomal abnormalities, such as Bloom, Fanconi, and Down syndromes. There is nothing in M.M.'s history that would indicate that she fits into any of these groups.

4. **e**   all of the above

Rationale

Statistical analysis has shown that several factors present at diagnosis are predictive of a more favorable prognosis. The single most important predictor is the histologic cell type. ALL has a significantly better prognosis than acute myelogenous leukemia (AML). Furthermore, among the subtypes of ALL, null cell with a positive CALLA reaction responds to therapy better than those with either B-cell or T-cell markers.

Children between the ages of 2 and 10 years have consistently better prognoses than those diagnosed before 2 or after 10 years. Initial white blood cell counts greater than 50,000 and presence of hepatosplenomegaly are both associated with a poorer diagnosis than children with normal, low, or slightly elevated white blood cell counts and no evidence of liver or spleen enlargement.

5. **a**   Different drugs exert their effects on cells during different phases of the life cycle of a cell

Rationale

Anticancer drugs exert their effects on cells at different phases of the cell life cycle. Some drugs are said to be cycle-specific, or cycle-dependent, because they kill cells in a specific cell phase, whereas other drugs are said to be cycle-nonspecific, or cycle-independent, because they destroy cells regardless of phase. For example, methotrexate destroys cells in the early G_1 phase and the S phase of DNA replication. Bleomycin works during the G_2 phase, as well as the mitosis phase. Cyclophosphamide is believed to be one of the cell cycle-independent drugs. There are presently no drugs that effect cells in the resting, G_0, phase.

With the understanding of the cell life cycle and the limitations of different chemotherapeutic agents, the necessity for giving several drugs (to destroy cells in as many phases as possible), and the need to repeat doses over time (to destroy cells as they emerge from the resting phase) becomes clearer.

6. **b**   a known side effect of the chemotherapy

Rationale

The vast majority of chemotherapeutic agents cause some degree of bone marrow depression. Since the erythrocytes, granulocytes, thrombocytes, and, to some extent, agranulocytes are believed to be formed in the myeloid tissue (red bone marrow), anything that causes bone marrow depression will result in a decreased production of the formed elements of the blood. Since complete cessation of production of the erythrocytes, granulocytes, and thrombocytes would be fatal, M.M.'s complete blood count, differential, and platelet counts are determined before each repeated dose of chemotherapy. If the erythrocytes or platelet counts are too low, transfusions are indicated. If the absolute neutrophil count is 200 mm³ or less, chemotherapy is withheld to give the bone marrow time to recover and produce cells again.

7. **c**   anemia, hemorrage and infection

Rationale

In leukemia, the proliferating leukemic cells compete with the formed elements of the blood for nutrients essential for metabolism. Once chemotherapy is started, the problem is compounded with additional chemotherapy side effects of bone marrow depression. The three major life-threatening complications are (1) anemia caused by decreased production of erythrocytes, (2) infections resulting from neutropenia (diminished numbers of neutrophils), and (3) bleeding tendencies caused by thrombocytopenia (decrease in number of circulating thrombocytes).

More children with ALL die of one of these complications of therapy than of the disease itself. The majority of nursing care during treatment centers around preventing and treating these three complications.

Disseminated Intravascular Coagulation (DIC) Caused by Septicemia

1. **c**   fibrin split products and fibrinogen

   Rationale
   Decreased fibrinogen levels, usually 100, are commonly seen in individuals with DIC. To substantiate the diagnosis, testing for fibrin split products in serum by immunoassay is necessary. Increased levels of fibrin split products are not specific for DIC but with increased prothrombin time, partial prothrombin time, and decreased fibrinogen and platelets diagnosis can be confirmed. Initially, red blood cell and hematocrit are not affected and are, therefore, not initially discriminating.

2. **a**   head trauma with ensuing shock

   Rationale
   Both head trauma and shock have been documented as precipitating factors for DIC. Blood transfusions can precipitate DIC if they are not cross-matched correctly. M.H.'s blood was correctly matched before transfusion. Other predisposing factors to DIC include cardiopulmonary bypass, burns, aneurysm, pulmonary embolism, childbirth (both complicated and uncomplicated), poisonous snake bites, malignancy, sepsis, and heat stroke.

3. **b**   microvascular thrombi and systemic bleeding

   Rationale
   As clotting factors are consumed by microvascular thrombi, a generalized decrease in clotting factors outside the microvasculature leads to hemorrhage. The by-products of fibrinolysis also act as anticoagulants and contribute to bleeding.

4. **d**   platelets and cryoprecipitate

   Rationale
   His circulating volume is within normal limits so he does not need volume replacement. He lacks clotting factors and platelets so these would be the expected treatment of choice at this point.

5. **c**   hang the drip because you know heparin therapy is used for life-threatening DIC

   Rationale
   Although controversial at this time, heparin drips are an accepted therapy in life-threatening DIC. The theory behind its use suggests that heparin inhibits coagulation, prevents thrombi in the microvasculature, and, consequently, preserves clotting factors for use in the general circulation.

6. **e**   all of the above

   Rationale
   The goals for nursing care for any individual with DIC are to monitor for signs of organ dysfunction caused by thrombi and to monitor and prevent bleeding. Thrombi in the microvasculature could cause organ dysfunction of any involved organ. Brain and renal function deterioration could be evidenced by a decreased level of consciousness or decreased urinary output. Intramuscular injection potentially could cause hemorrhage because of the lack of clotting factors and should be prevented. As individuals with DIC are at risk for hemorrhage, the nurse must monitor the individual closely for any bleeding in an effort to prevent major hemorrhage. Signs of internal bleeding would be picked up by monitoring venous pressures.

16 Hemophilia A

1. **a**   iron deficiency anemia

   Rationale
   Iron deficiency anemia is the least likely possibility considering the normal blood work results and unremarkable skin findings (other than bruising). Any child who is seen with multiple ecchymoses and hematomas should be considered an abuse victim until proved otherwise. The extent of J.B.'s visible ecchymoses indicates trauma that predated his current accident. Leukemia is a less likely possibility, in light of his normal complete blood count and differential. But bruising can be one of the first visible indicators of leukemia. Hemophilia should be highly suspect because of the excessive bleeding from his sutured laceration, oozing abrasions, multiple ecchymoses and hematoma, history of easy bruising, and increased bleeding after circumcision.

2. **b**   type A (classic) hemophilia

   Rationale
   Classic hemophilia is characterized by abnormalities in partial prothrombin time and clotting factor VIII, a component of the intrinsic coagulation pathway. Individuals with this disorder have normal vasculature, platelets, and fibrinogen levels, and all clotting factors are normal except factor VIII. Christmas disease is another name for hemophilia type B, or factor IX deficiency. Von Willebrand disease presents with abnormalities of both factor VIII and platelets. Given the abnormal clotting study findings and lack of evidence of recent or remote fractures, the likelihood of child abuse is significantly diminished.

3. **d** All of the above

Rationale

The solution to this question can be easily visualized with pedigree charts, as shown here.

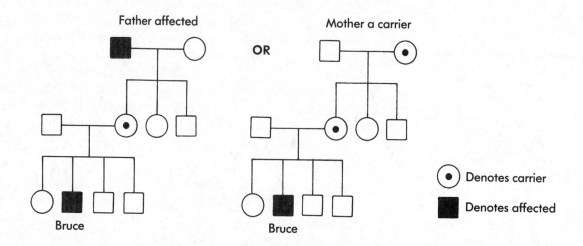

Father affected   OR   Mother a carrier

Bruce

Bruce

⊙ Denotes carrier

■ Denotes affected

Classic hemophilia is transmitted as an X-linked recessive disorder and always affects males who are homozygous for the trait. Therefore, all the sons of a male hemophiliac will be normal, whereas all daughters will be obligate carriers. Male offspring of a carrier have a 50% chance of having the disease, female offspring have a 50% chance of being carriers. Research has indicated that all members of a particular family will have similar clinical severity of the disease. Carriers do have lower levels of factor VIII than the normal population. These women are occasionally noted to bleed more than the average during menstruation or childbirth, but this is rarely a significant problem for them.

4. **c** Mild

Rationale

Severity of hemophilia is based on the assayed level of factor VIII in the blood. Severe is less than 1%, moderate is 1%, mild is 5% to 50%. Thirty percent is the minimal level of factor VIII necessary for effective hemostasis. It is interesting to note that individuals with mild or moderately severe hemophilia may not be detected until they undergo surgery or sustain major trauma.

5. **a**   packed cells

   Rationale

   Packed cells contain only red blood cells. The plasma portion that contains factor VIII has been removed during the centrifugation process. Fresh frozen plasma will replace all clotting factors except platelets. This was the mainstay of replacement therapy for hemophiliacs in the 1950s and 1960s. Unfortunately transfusion reactions and plasma volume overload were significant complications of this therapy, and its use was restricted to hospital settings. In 1965, J.G. Pool discovered that cryoprecipitate, a factor VIII rich portion, could be separated from plasma. This product eliminated the problem of volume overload, since it comprised a small volume compared to the total plasma fraction. Koate is a commercially available lyophilized preparation of pure factor VIII.

6. **e**   all of the above

   Rationale

   Anaphylaxis or allergic reactions and post-transfusion hemolysis are less common with concentrate therapy than when nonpurified blood products are given. Diphenhydramine hydrochloride (Benadryl) can be taken 1/2 hour before concentrate therapy by individuals with known mild allergic reactions. Hepatitis and AIDS are potentially fatal complications that may arise from using blood products obtained from pooled donors. The causative factors in AIDS remain unspecified. However, the possibility of developing AIDS is greater after use of the lyophilized concentrates than of cryoprecitpitate or fresh frozen plasma.

7. **d**   a multidisciplinary team of caregivers

   Rationale

   In 1975, Congress established a Hemophilia Diagnostic and Treatment Center Program. Various medical centers across the United States were designated as specialized for hemophilia care. At that time, the recommendation was for care by a multidisciplinary team to include physicians of various specialties, nurses, social workers, physiotherapists, genetic counselors, nutritionists, and collectors of data from all caregivers.

8. **b**   hemarthroses with joint destruction

   Rationale

   Joint damage from frequent, recurrent bleeds is the primary cause of morbidity. Individuals often have premonitory symptoms of warmth or prickling at the onset of a bleed and should begin replacement therapy immediately. Since the onset of home treatment with concentrates, morbidity from joint damage has decreased significantly. Muscle spasms, gastrointestinal bleeds, and hematuria are problems encountered, but less often than hemarthroses. Chronic renal failure is rare. Intracranial bleeding usually occurs after trauma rather than spontaneously but can be a significant cause of mortality if undetected. All hemophiliacs who sustain head trauma should be evaluated and treated immediately and need instruction for careful follow-up. An interesting finding is the fact that hemophilic children often have abnormal electroencephalograms, suggesting possible previous subclinical bleeds with cortical scarring.

9. **f**   all of the above

Rationale

Plasmapheresis can provide temporary hemostasis if it is followed immediately by infusion of factor VII, when the antibody (inhibitor) levels are lowest. Unfortunately, the antibody levels tend to reappear rather rapidly. It is not well understood why giving factor IX would help an individual with a factor VIII deficiency, but 50% of the individuals with inhibitors can be successfully managed by factor IX replacement. It is felt that giving the activated prothrombin complex (factor IX) would bypass the site of action of the factor VIII inhibitor and allow subsequent clotting steps to proceed. Fifteen percent of individuals with factor VIII deficiency develop inhibitors; less than that number of factor IX deficient individuals develop inhibitors. FEIBA is a relatively new compound that seems to have antibody-bypassing activity, though its active principle has eluded investigators. The use of steroids is not highly recommended but could be helpful in some cases. Administration of large doses of factor VIII, in spite of factor VIII antibodies, is helpful in life-threatening bleeds.

10. **a**   heparin

Rationale

Aspirin, indomethacin (Indocin), phenylbutazone (Butazolidin), and antiallergy medication (Chlor Trimeton) all inhibit platelet aggregation and prolong bleeding. Heparin is also a potent anticoagulant. Small amounts of heparin are frequently added to factor IX concentrates to inhibit thromboplastic activity. Factor IX deficient individuals with liver dysfunction may develop thromboses from factor IX replacement (prothrombin complex) without heparin.

11. **c**   Diphtheria, pertussis, tetanus (DPT) and measles, mumps, and rubella (MMR) immunizations are contraindicated

Rationale

Although intramuscular and subcutaneous injections should be avoided for all hemophiliacs, it is recommended that children receive these basic immunization series. Acetaminophen may be utilized for postinjection discomfort. Obesity and snow and water skiing put increased stress on joints that are already increasingly vulnerable to bleeding. Post-tonsillitis hemorrhage is common, and blood accumulation could be visually mistaken for mumps if allowed to progress. Factor VIII (or IX) therapy is mandatory before any invasive procedure.

Hypertension Leading to Congestive Heart Failure (CHF)

1. **a**   high potassium intake

   Rationale
   High potassium intake is not currently implicated as a cause of essential hypertension. There is evidence that it may be protective. High sodium intake, genetic factors, and sympathetic nervous system activity have all been implicated as playing a role in the development of essential hypertension.

2. **d**   Afterload becomes so high that the ventricles cannot maintain adequate forward flow

   Rationale
   Current research indicates that congestive heart failure associated with hypertension is the result of increased systemic vascular resistance, producing increased afterload. The left ventricle initially compensates by hypertrophic enlargement. Eventually, the afterload may elevate to levels the ventricle cannot overcome, even with its increased size. Preload is usually unaltered or slightly increased. Structural changes in the cardiac valves may occur as a result of ventricular hypertrophy or dilation, but this is not regarded as the cause of the congestive heart failure.

3. **a** Loss of synchronized atrial and ventricular contraction resulted in mild pulmonary edema

Rationale

Loss of synchronized atrial and ventricular contraction has been shown to reduce cardiac output by 20% to 50%. The venous and pulmonary beds then must store the blood not moving forward. As the pulmonary capillary hydrostatic pressures rise, fluid is forced out of the lung capillaries into the interstitial spaces and into the alveoli. The fluid in the alveoli slows oxygen diffusion. The individual experiences shortness of breath as the respiratory center responds to this hypoxemia. Individuals in this situation are usually anxious and experience sympathetic response; however, it is not the primary cause of their dyspnea. An enlarged left atrium may displace the bronchi and/or the esophagus. Individuals who sense this anatomical change usually complain of dysphagia rather than dyspnea.

4. **d** Blood flow was not turbulent enough to make sounds

Rationale

Measurement of blood pressure by cuff depends on the cuff to produce restricted flow and turbulence in the artery; this is heard as Korotkoff sounds. In many individuals with hypertension, flow is not turbulent enough to produce sound in the upper systolic region. The resulting silence is termed the auscultatory gap. Although no sounds are heard, the pulse can be palpated during the gap. Therefore, the correct technique of indirect blood pressure measurement includes palpating the systolic pressure before listening for the Korotkoff sounds. This ensures that the true systolic pressure will be measured.

5. **c** incomplete emptying of ventricles

Rationale

The only heart sounds usually heard in healthy adults are S_1 and S_2. These represent the closure of the atrioventricular (A-V) and semilunar valves. When "gallop" sounds are heard, they almost always indicate pathology in adults. Mrs. B.'s gallop is the sound of blood being ejected into her overfilled ventricles during atrial systole. Her ventricular walls have also become noncompliant as a result of hypertrophy and volume overload; thus, the blood "thuds" against these walls during ventricular filling.

6. **c** It acts directly on vascular smooth muscle

Rationale

The exact mechanism for vasodilatation is still unclear, but some actions have been shown to play no role. Nitroprusside does not act through the adrenergic system. At the present time, research indicates that nitroprusside is effective in lowering blood pressure and vascular resistance by direct stimulation of the smooth muscle of arteries and veins, causing them to dilate.

Myocardial Infarction (MI) Caused by Coronary Artery Occlusion

1. **b, c**   essential hypertension and smoking

   Rationale
   Age, male sex, and family history of early cardiac death are all significant risk factors; however, they are not alterable. Cigarette smoking and elevated blood pressure are currently considered to be both significant and alterable. The rate of the atherosclerotic process is slowed and the incidence of myocardial infarction reduced when cigarette smoking is discontinued. The incidence of myocardial infarction is also reduced when hypertension is controlled by a therapeutic regimen.

2. **a**   lipid deposition in the tunica intima

   Rationale
   In simplest terms, atherosclerosis is a condition in which vessel walls thicken and harden. These changes occur when fat and fibrin deposits inside the arteries harden over time.

   One of the earliest events is the laying down of lipids in the innermost layer of a vessel, the tunica intima. The so-called fatty streaks are smooth muscle cells filled with lipids. They form along the tunica intima but do not occlude the artery. These fatty streaks are known to be present even in childhood.

   In time the fatty streak become a fibrous plaque as a result of cellular proliferation, accumulation of fat, and formation of connective tissue. It protrudes into the vessel lumen and may invade deeper into the vessel wall. Some fibrous plaques eventually calcify and cause the vessel surface to ulcerate.

3. **b**   complete occlusion of a coronary artery that produces myocardial ischemia for 1 hour or more

Rationale
Current research indicates that myocardial cell death and necrosis (infarction) result when occlusion of a coronary artery deprives the myocardium of oxygen for at least 1 hour. Dysrhythmias, in which atrial and ventricular synchronization is lost, may reduce cardiac output enough to cause myocardial ischemia. However, the probability that myocardial infarction will result is remote. Coronary artery narrowing usually does not produce symptoms until the lumen is less than 70% of the original diameter. Many individuals develop compensatory collateral circulation as the athersclerotic plaque progresses and do not become symptomatic until the arterial lumen is stenosed by 95% or more. Structural changes in the cardiac valves do produce abnormal hemodynamics, and the cardiac output can be restricted enough to produce myocardial ischemia. The end stage of untreated valve disease may demonstrate extremely low cardiac outputs that are inadequate for myocardial perfusion. Myocardial infarction may result, but this is rarely the cause of myocardial infarction.

4. **a**   myocardial ischemia

Rationale
The typical chest pain of myocardial infarction is considered to be referred pain originating from myocardial ischemia. There are two current theories used to explain this mechanism. The ischemic theory proposes that the pain is referred pain that results from stimulation of pain fibers located in the coronary arteries by a hypothetical "P" substance. The P substance has not been identified but is thought to be lactic acid and/or bradykinin released from myocardial cells with anaerobic metabolism. The tension-mechanical theory proposes that the pain results from stimulation of the sympathetic nerve endings located in the coronary arteries that respond to stretch or tension. Most individuals with a history of cardiac pain are found to have a coronary arterial thrombus at autopsy. Sensory fibers from the heart enter the spinal cord at the same level as sensory fibers from the cutaneous vessels of the chest and arms. The pattern of pain referral is believed to result from brain interpretation and integration of incoming stimuli from the cardiac vessels as originating in the cutaneous vessels. The other responses are not known to cause chest pain directly.

5. **d** left ventricular dysfunction

Rationale

Myocardial ischemia, injury, and infarction all cause dysfunction of the left ventricular myocardium that is related to the location and size of the hypoxic tissue. Because Mr. G.'s infarct was anterior and produced electrocardiographic changes in the first four chest leads, he undoubtedly had some degree of left ventricular dysfunction. Left ventricular dysfunction reduces the stroke volume because the hypoxia decreases contractility. If the cardiac rate and systemic vascular resistance are unchanged, the reduced stroke volume will result in reduced cardiac output and lowered arterial blood pressure. Increased venous return to the left atrium might cause an elevated pulmonary capillary wedge pressure. However, with normal left ventricular function, the arterial pressure would be expected to remain the same or to be elevated. Decreased left ventricular afterload would result from arterial vasodilatation and decreased systemic vascular resistance. The arterial blood pressure might drop if no compensatory changes in cardiac output were made, but the pulmonary capillary wedge pressure would be expected to remain the same or decrease. Hypovolemia would be expected to cause lowered right atrial and pulmonary capillary wedge pressures.

6. **c** It prevents further thrombosis by interfering with conversion of prothrombin to thrombin

Rationale

Heparin interferes with conversion of prothrombin to thrombin. At therapeutic levels of administration, this prevents further thrombus formation. Heparin does not alter the structure or existing thrombi, nor does it affect vitamin K metabolism.

1. **c**   decreased contractility

Rationale

Ejection fraction (EF) is the percentage of total ventricular blood volume that is ejected during each contraction (stroke volume divided by end-diastolic volume). As such, EF is an index of left ventricular function. EF is normally 50% to 70% of ventricular blood volume because the ventricles do not totally empty with each contraction. Mr. B.'s EF is markedly diminished. This is characteristic of alcoholic cardiomyopathy, as well as other forms of congestive cardiomyopathy. There are several factors that seem to contribute to this decreased EF. First, alcohol appears to have a direct toxic effect on the heart, reducing its ability to contract. Several studies have demonstrated a significant reduction in EF in individuals with a history of significant alcohol consumption but who otherwise have normal electrocardiograms and normal cardiothoracic ratios on chest roentgenogram. In later stages the heart dilates and myocardial contractility is further reduced. At autopsy the nonspecific pathological findings in the myocardial wall include areas of patchy fibrosis, various degrees of muscle fiber degeneration, and even some hypertrophied muscle fibers. Extensive mitrochodrial degeneration is also noted by electron microscopy. This disruption of the energy-producing structures probably contributes to diminished contractility.

    The amount of alcohol required to reduce contractility and/or produce ventricular dilatation is not known. It is probable that some individuals are more sensitive than others. Alcoholics who show a predilection for cardiac damage constitute a separate group from those who develop liver damage. Treatment of congestive heart failure caused by alcohol induced cardiomyopathy is ineffective unless total abstinence from alcohol is part of the treatment plan.

2. **d**   all of the above

Rationale

The hemodynamic changes seen in congestive cardiomyopathy are those of pump failure. The stroke volume is reduced in the early stage of cardiomyopathy. However, this may be compensated for by an increased heart rate that results in an adequate cardiac output. The heart is, however, unable to increase heart rate enough during exercise, causing an increase in end-diastolic pressure of the left ventricle and dyspnea.

The minute volume is diminished as well as the stroke volume in later stages of cardiomyopathy. The ventricles dilate as a result of increasing end-systolic volume; even if the ventricles are dilated for a long time the individual may be asymptomatic. This is because, within physiological limits, increased ventricular volume results in stretching of the ventricular fibers, causing them to contract more forcefully, resulting in an increased stroke volume (Starling's law). This process is very dependent on blood volume; therefore, diuretics should be carefully balanced at this stage. If the individual has too much circulating blood volume, the physiologic limits will be exceeded. If the individual is significantly hypovolemic, however, the end-diastolic volume may be diminished, resulting in decreased stroke volume. The disadvantage of dilatation soon overtakes the advantages as the individual moves into the decompensation phase. According to La Place's law, dilatation is accompanied by greater wall tension and pressure that increases myocardial oxygen consumption. Digoxin, a commonly used positive inotropic agent, is frequently used. Digoxin markedly increases the force of myocardial contraction and causes the stroke volume to increase. The disadvantage of this particular medication is that it also markedly increases myocardial oxygen consumption. A combination of physiologic compensatory mechanisms and medical therapeutics can maintain cardiac function for a variable period of time. This type of cardiomyopathy, unfortunately, generally results in a progressive deterioration in cardiac function. Mr. B.'s fatigue is a direct result of this decreased cardiac function.

3. **c**   prevent thrombus formation within the chambers of the dilated heart

Rationale

In dilated congestive cardiomyopathy, the ventricular dilatation is associated with poor ventricular contraction that, in turn, results in a low ejection fraction and large end-systolic volumes. The latter seems to limit atrial emptying, which in turn leads to high atrial end-diastolic volume with resulting dilatation. Thrombi (blood clots) frequently form in one or both atrial appendages as a result of poor atrial emptying and relative stasis of blood. The large end-systolic ventricular volume causes relative stasis of blood in the apical portions of the ventricular cavities and results in intracavitary thrombi. These intracavitary thrombi have the potential to give rise to pulmonary or systemic emboli that may be life-threatening. For this reason, individuals are given prophylactic anticoagulant therapy.

4. a   the valvular regurgitation is caused by papillary muscle dysfunction

Rationale

The leaflets of the cardiac valves are usually normal unless there is other underlying pathology such as rheumatic heart disease. Occasionally the margin of the mitral and tricuspid valves is thickened by fibrous tissue. The latter is more common in individuals who have had atrioventricular valve regurgitation for a long time. This thickening appears to result from regurgitation and does not by itself cause incompetence. The cause of valvular regurgitation in Mr. B. appears to be papillary muscle dysfunction, because the tricuspid and mitral valve annuli are usually only mildly dilated. The papillary muscles are muscle bundles that are situated parallel to the ventricular walls and extend from the walls to the chordae tendineae. The chordae tendineae connect the papillary muscles to the valve leaflets. Dysfunction of the papillary muscle, as is commonly seen in cardiomyopathy, interferes with the function of the valve leaflets and allows the valves to prolapse into the atrial chambers during ventricular contraction, leading to regurgitation.

5. b   myocardial muscle disease

Rationale

The primary reason for dysrhythmias in cardiomyopathy is that the muscle is diseased. The myocardium is hypertrophied in part and the ventricles are generally dilated in the later stages. The stretching effects of these changes cause irritability. Individuals with cardiomyopathy are not, however, restricted to ventricular dysrhythmias. Because cardiomyopathy affects almost every aspect of cardiac function, individuals commonly have atrial dysrhythmias, such as atrial fibrillation, and intraventricular conduction defects, such as bundle branch block. Mr. B.'s electrocardiogram demonstrated left bundle branch block in addition to ventricular hypertrophy and atrial enlargement. Most of these possible causes may contribute to his dysrhythmias.

1. **b**   excessive loss of blood and fluids

    Rationale
    Hypovolemia is the result of a loss of blood and fluid with a resulting deficit in the intravascular volume. Because the pelvis is a vascular area and Mr. C. suffered multiple pelvic fractures, an initial amount of blood loss is reflected in these injuries. More significant, however, is the ruptured spleen, which accounts for major blood loss. The spleen can store several liters of blood at any given time. The collection of blood in the retroperitoneal space is indeed inaccessible. However, it collects there because of the nature of the internal injuries.

2. **a**   increased heart rate and oliguria

    Rationale
    The increased heart rate is a compensatory mechanism that attempts to maintain normal cardiac output by increasing the number of times the heart ejects a stroke volume per minute. When the need to maintain blood pressure is sensed, the heart rate increases in an effort to pump more blood to the vital organs. The initial increase in rate is usually effective, but as the circulating volume continues to decrease, the increased rate is no longer sufficient.

    Decreased urine output and decreased available fluid in tissues also represent compensatory mechanisms. Urine output decreases as aldosterone and antidiuretic hormone (ADH) are secreted, producing body water conservation. Aldosterone is secreted from the adrenal cortex, causing sodium and water retention in the kidney. The ADH secreted from the anterior pituitary also assists in maintaining adequate blood volume.

3. **c**   secretion of epinephrine and norepinephrine in response to decreased blood pressure

   Rationale
   In early stages of shock, baroreceptors located in the aortic arch sense a decrease in mean arterial blood pressure. In response, epinephrine and norepinephrine are secreted into the blood stream. Results of actions include α-adrenergic and β-adrenergic responses. An α-adrenergic response includes increased blood pressure as a result of arterial vasoconstriction, diversion of blood to vital organs, and decreased venous capacitance. β-Adrenergic response results in increased heart rate and contractility.

4. **b**   decreased tissue perfusion

   Rationale
   A dramatic decrease in circulating blood volume results in decreased oxygenation of tissues. This can be seen from Mr. C.'s PO_2 level of 41 mmHg. As the blood volume decreases, the tissues are not being adequately oxygenated. C.C.'s respiratory rate increased to 46 as he tried to compensate for this hypoxic state. Hypoxia can lead to metabolic acidosis if oxygen levels are not corrected because of the buildup of carbon dioxide. In addition, high PCO_2 levels trigger increased respirations. Mr. C. was started on oxygen, which decreased his respiratory rate to 28 and increased his PO_2 level to 84 mm Hg, which is now in the low normal range.

5. **d**   compensatory mechanism in response to stress

   Rationale
   When the body perceives an injury, it reacts in a number of ways. The stress response activates the adrenal medulla to release epinephrine. Epinephrine increases blood glucose by increasing glycogenolysis and gluconeogenesis in the liver, while inhibiting glycogen synthesis. Epinephrine also decreases insulin release from the pancreas. Mr. C.'s body is responding to this injury by trying to resist its effects.

Ventricular Septal Defect (VSD)

1. **b**   congestive heart failure

   Rationale
   The higher oxygen saturation in the right ventricle relative to the right atrium indicates that saturated blood is entering the right ventricle from the left ventricle through the VSD. The oxygen saturation would normally be the same in both the right atrium and the right ventricle and would be lower than that in the left ventricle. In addition, the oxygen saturation in the left ventricle is equal to that in the left atrium, indicating that no saturated blood is moving from the right ventricle to the left ventricle. Since no desaturated blood is moving through the VSD from right to left and, hence, into the systemic circulation, the shunt is not the cause of A.B.'s cyanosis. However, A.B. does have congestive heart failure as evidenced by his failure to thrive, diaphoresis, fatigue, and tachycardia. It is also well documented that decreased cardiac output can cause cyanosis because less oxygen is reaching peripheral tissues. Congestive heart failure causes decreased cardiac output and is the cause of A.B.'s cyanosis.

2. **c**   mother's age

   Rationale
   In general, little is known about the relation of the father's age to the incidence of VSD. Though many studies of siblings with congenital heart defects (CHDs) have shown an increased incidence among siblings, this has yet to be demonstrated among cousins. Likewise a family history of high blood pressure has not been associated with an increase in the incidence of VSD. Advanced maternal age has been linked to an increase in the incidence of VSD. Note that this is based on what is *currently known* about the incidence of CHD within families. It may be that the other factors presented as alternatives are in some way related to the incidence of VSD, but these connections have yet to be established in

the literature.

3. **d**   relative difference between pulmonary and systemic resistance

Rationale

With a large VSD the pressures within the two ventricles are equal at systemic levels because blood flow is basically unimpeded across the opening. Pressure differences are usually the first determinant of shunt direction; however, in A.B.'s case this would not be true. This makes his shunt a dependent shunt; that is, the relative differences in A.B.'s pulmonary and systemic vascular resistances determine the direction of blood flow through his VSD. The results of his catheterization reveal that his systemic resistance is greater than his pulmonary resistance, so blood flows from left to right through the VSD. This is because systemic resistance is reflected by the left side of the heart, whereas pulmonary resistance is reflected by the right side of the heart. A further clue is that oxygen saturation is higher in the right ventricle than in the right atrium; this also indicates that oxygenated blood is flowing through the VSD from the left ventricle to the right ventricle.

4. **d**   Pulmonary and systemic resistance were equal

Rationale

There is an immediate drop in pulmonary vascular resistance at birth, as well as a rise in systemic vascular resistance. Nonetheless pulmonary vascular resistance requires several weeks to decrease to normal levels. Immediately after birth there may not be enough difference between pulmonary vascular resistance and systemic vascular resistance to push any blood through the VSD. Thus the murmur was not apparent at that time. As soon as systemic vascular resistance exceeds pulmonary vascular resistance, blood would move through the VSD and create a murmur.

5. **b**   direction of blood flow through VSD

Rationale

The blood flow through A.B.'s VSD has reversed and is now flowing from right to left. The higher oxygen saturation in the left atrium relative to the left ventricle demonstrates that saturated blood is entering the left ventricle from the right ventricle. Since this puts desaturated blood from the right side of the heart into the systemic circulation through the left ventricle and aorta, A.B. has systemically decreased oxygen saturation, which manifests as cyanosis. The shunt reversal is caused by irreversible changes that have taken place in A.B.'s pulmonary vasculature.

In response to the increased blood volume in the lungs, the muscle layer of the pulmonary arterioles has increased and extended farther into the small vessels. Proliferation of the intimal layer of these arterioles has also occurred. In vessels such as arterioles, when the length of the tube remains constant and the viscosity of the blood flowing through it remains fairly constant, any changes in resistance will be caused by changes in the radius of the tube (Poiseuille's Law). Because of the increased muscle layer and intimal proliferation, the diameter of the arteriolar opening is smaller; thus the resistance is increased. Overall this creates increased pulmonary vascular resistance. In the event that pulmonary vascular resistance exceeds systemic vascular resistance, blood flow will go from right to left through the VSD. This phenomenon, known as Eisenmenger syndrome, is a late complication of VSD.

1. **e**   a, b

   Rationale

   In emphysema the elastin and fiber network within the alveoli becomes damaged. The alveoli have a tendency to become larger, and thus the walls of the alveoli break down. This results in larger air spaces, creating a reduction in the alveolar diffusing surface. Because the walls of the alveoli are destroyed, the lungs become more compliant (distensible) as a result of a loss in the muscle and fibrous tissue. Elastic recoil is also lost, therefore causing air to become trapped. This air trapping increases the size of the airway during inspiration, and on expiration collapse of the small airways occurs. Therefore, it is common to see a prolongation in the forced expiratory volume (FEV), a decrease in tidal volume (TV), and an increase in total lung capacity (TLC).

2. **c**   hyperinflation of the lungs

   Rationale

   Hyperinflation of the lungs causes the anteroposterior chest diameter to increase, giving rise to the "barrel chest" appearance of emphysema. The chest tends to become fixed in the inspiratory position. Other manifestations include prominent anterior chest and dorsal kyphosis. The elevated rib margin seen in these individuals is caused by the trapping of air, resulting in lung enlargement and inability to recoil effectively. The accessory muscles of respiration are used to help raise the thorax on inspiration, and the abdominal muscles are used with expiration to help force the air out of the lungs.

3. **c**   hypoventilation

Rationale

Retention of carbon dioxide in the lungs is common in emphysema as a result of hypoventilation in relation to an uneven matching of ventilation and perfusion. Carbon dixoide is not adequately excreted and, therefore, builds up in the lungs. This increase in carbon dioxide causes the ventilatory rate to increase. However, when the disease becomes severe, the increase in the ventilation rate does not help return the PCO_2 to normal. When retention of the carbon dioxide becomes chronic, the medullary chemoreceptor becomes depressed. Therefore, the person may lose the stimulus for breathing that is driven by increased carbon dioxide. He or she must then rely on the peripheral chemoreceptors for the stimulation of breathing. With the retention of carbon dioxide, the decrease in pH is counteracted by the renal system through the retention of bicarbonate. Therefore, most individuals have a *compensated respiratory acidosis*. Hence, hypercarbia and acidemia cause a shift to the right on the oxyhemoglobin dissociation curve because these factors have a tendency to reduce the affinity of the hemoglobin for oxygen.

4. **b**   low concentration

Rationale

As discussed, the individual with emphysema derives the stimulus for breathing from the peripheral chemoreceptors located in the carotid arteries and on the arch of the aorta. Because these sites are sensitive to a decrease in oxygen, oxygen administration may tend to decrease this stimulus, resulting in respiratory failure and hypoventilation. Therefore, oxygen has to be administered in a low concentration (25% to 35%) and at a low flow rate (1 to 2 L/min) to prevent carbon dioxide narcosis. This is because the individual depends on hypoxia as the major stimulus for breathing. If too high a concentration of oxygen is given to the individual, the hypoxic drive to breathe is eliminated.

5. **b**   COPD increases the body's need for calories

Rationale

Malnutrition is a common finding in individuals with advancing COPD. It happens for a variety of reasons, but among the most important of these is the effect of the increased work of breathing. The individual must use the accessory muscles of respiration continuously to raise the thorax, as well as the abdominal muscles, to force exhalation. This increased work takes more energy in the form of calories. Individuals with emphysema can use more than 700 calories/day just for breathing. In addition, the appetite is often decreased from fatigue and as a side effect of medications. Dyspnea itself makes eating very difficult even if appetite is present. Thus in the individual with COPD weight loss results from a combination of increased energy requirements and decreased intake.

Bronchopneumonia in the Elderly

1. **b**   infection

   Rationale
   Mr. B.'s hypertension appears to be under control with his medication (142/80). Diabetes is not likely to be the cause because blood sugar is 140 mg. It is not unusual for the elderly to have increased blood sugar as part of normal aging (normal range is 80 to 120 mg for young adults). Mr. B.'s history, so far, is not indicative of a failure-to-thrive syndrome. Respiratory infections in the elderly produce metabolic stress but often do not manifest themselves initially with typical symptoms seen in the younger individual, such as fever, cough, chills, pleural pain, and hemoptysis. Minor changes in the functional status of the elderly may indicate a rapidly progressing infection. Common infections in the elderly involve the urinary tract and the respiratory tract. Mr. B.'s laboratory data do not indicate a urinary tract infection since the urinalysis revealed normal results. Therefore, it is likely that he has a respiratory infection, given his recent history.

2. **b**   Fever, tachycardia, and increased respirations are often not present

   Rationale
   Several changes in the aging lung contribute to the atypical presentation of pneumonia in Mr. B. Among these are decreased alveolar surface area for gas exchange, decreased air flow rate, and decreased oxygen tension. Normal Pao_2 in a 20-year-old is about 90, whereas that in a 70-year-old is about 70. The body's responses to hypercapnea (increased carbon dioxide) and hypoxia (decreased oxygen) are lessened. Thus the usual response to a relative lack of oxygen brought on by pneumonia (increased respirations, increased heart rate, and increased blood pressure) may not be seen in the elderly until the illness is well advanced.

Fever is a normal part of the body's immune response to infection. This immune response is slower in the elderly so fever may not appear early in pneumonia. Loss of appetite, lethargy, and changes in functional and mental status are often more useful than changes in vital signs in the early diagnosis of respiratory infection in the elderly.

3. **a**   hydration and chest physiotherapy

Rationale

One of the most important body defenses against respiratory illness is the mucociliary system. Cilia line 80% of the central airways and move in coordinated waves to clear particles and microorganisms from the airways. They can normally move mucus and trapped particles toward the pharynx at the rate of 10 to 20 mm/min.

Elderly persons experience significant changes in this system, including decreases in both number and activity of cilia. In addition, the cough mechanism decreases in force, volume, and rate. The overall effect of these changes is decreased ability to clear inhaled particles from the tracheobronchial tree. If the elderly person has a chronic pulmonary condition along with an acute infection, the problems are compounded. Hydration and chest physiotherapy are very useful in loosening and clearing pulmonary secretions.

4. **b**   *Streptococcus pneumoniae* in his lungs

Rationale

Although sputum color is not absolutely diagnostic of a particular bacterium, it can be helpful in supporting such a diagnosis. Infection by *S. pneumoniae* produces rusty sputum, whereas *Pseudomonas aeruginosa* produces green sputum. In addition to color, sputum cultures and Gram's stain identify the causative agent, if it is bacterial.

5. **d**   all of the above

Rationale

Sepsis is a serious consequence of infection in the elderly. It is a higher risk for them because diagnosis of infection may be delayed as a result of atypical presentation. The atypical presentation, in turn, is caused by the slower immune and respiratory responses of elderly adults. In addition, decreased pulmonary clearance slows the removal of bacteria and debris from the respiratory system. All of these factors combine to allow the bacteria more time in which to grow and spread to the blood stream, as well as to provide an excellent growth medium in unexpectorated respiratory secretions.

6. **d**   Have influenza immunization every year and pneumococcal immunization every 5 years

Rationale

Annual influenza immunization is recommended for adults over the age of 65 by the Center for Disease Control (CDC). Pneumococcal immunization every 5 years is currently recommended. It should be administered to the elderly, especially those over 65, with chronic diseases or immunosuppression.

1. **c**   family genetic pedigree

   Rationale
   CF is inherited. Both parents carry the gene and will pass the disease on to one of four of their offspring. It is an autosomal recessive trait; this means that there is a 25% risk that each pregnancy will produce a child who has the disease, a 50% risk that each pregnancy will produce a child who carries the disease trait, and a 25% chance that each pregnancy will produce a child who neither has or carries the disease. CF affects the exocrine secretory glands and cells. Serous secretions are concentrated; mucous secretions are thick and tenacious. CF affects the respiratory system and, in the majority of cases, the pancreatic system.

2. **d**   all of the above

   Rationale
   The primary cause of malnutrition in individuals with CF is their malabsorption of fats and protein and deficiency of fat-soluble vitamins. It has also been documented that individuals with CF use more calories to breathe, clear secretions, and participate in daily activities than " normal" individuals. The majority of children with CF have pancreatic involvement. The pancreatic enzymes are necessary for digestion/absorption of food, and these enzymes are not available to or are limited in availability to the child with pancreatic CF. Enzymes produced in the pancreas are prevented from moving out of the pancreas by thick secretions that block pancreatic ducts. The blockage of the ducts leads to eventual fibrotic changes in the pancreas.

3. **b** to break the infectious process

Rationale

To stop the infectious process, prevent further lung damage, and to reduce mucus production. When the individual becomes infected, pulmonary mucus production is increased. The mucus provides a medium for bacterial growth, which leads to increased mucus production and increased blockage of the respiratory tract. The blockage allows mucus to sit in the lung, thereby encouraging bacteria to grow, and the process is cyclical unless it can be stopped by the use of antibiotics.

4. **d** a, c

Rationale

In the lungs, the thickened secretions lead to blocked bronchioles and subsequent emphysematic changes. The thick secretions are a medium for bacterial growth, which in turn leads to increased secretions and development of further respiratory deterioration. Chest physiotherapy is used to loosen secretions and to facilitate their movement from the lungs to be expectorated. Removal of secretions facilitates air exchange by removing a mechanical block (secretions) to air exchange. Chest physiotherapy may be performed five or more times a day along with postural drainage. Aerosol treatments using bronchodilators and mucolytics may be used to help loosen secretions and open airways to facilitate air exchange.

5. **d** all of the above

Rationale

S.S. will probably experience periodic bacterial respiratory infections with increased airway blockage and emphysematic changes. Respiratory effort will become more difficult. She can expect increased oxygen requirements, increasing dyspnea, and development of a barrel chest. S.S. will continue to have malabsorption problems and will need to continue enzyme replacement and vitamin supplements. A high-calorie diet with high-calorie supplements will be indicated for the duration of her life. She is at risk for meconium ileus equivalent, which may lead to partial or complete bowel obstruction. There is also risk of development of liver disease, though the risk varies among individuals. Damage is caused by blockage of the bile ducts and eventual fibrotic changes in the liver, which are followed by cirrhosis and portal hypertension.

6. **f** a, b, c

Rationale

Pulmonary hypertension, secondary to obstructive respiratory diasease, may lead to right-sided heart failure and ultimately is the cause of death of many children with CF.

1. **c** positive familial history

   Rationale
   Positive family history is the most significant factor in a positive diagnosis of asthma. Asthma appears to be genetically transmitted, although the mechanism for this transmission is not clearly understood. Children tend to develop asthmatic symptoms before the fifth birthday, and D. fits this pattern. Gender also seems to be a factor in that twice as many boys as girls develop asthma in childhood. Eczema is common in children with asthma but has not been causally linked to development of childhood asthma at this time. There is no suggestion in the past history that D.'s growth pattern is a cause of concern.

2. **b** IgG

   Rationale
   IgG antibodies are formed in reaction to an antigen's entering the body and creating an immune response. The immune response precipitates the release of mediators from the mast cells in the bronchial epithelium. These mediators include bronchospasm, mucous membrane edema, and increased mucus production. This antigen-antibody response can result in airway obstruction and hypoxia.

3. **a** dyspnea and wheezing

   Rationale
   Both dyspnea and wheezing are the result of airway obstruction. As edema and mucus block the airways, air becomes trapped, causing an increase in the expiratory phase of respiration. In an effort to compensate for airway obstruction and need for oxygen, children increase their rate of respiration. This ventilation/ perfusion mismatch leads to hypoxia and buildup of carbon dioxide as oxygen saturation falls off. Wheezes are high-pitched, musical sounds that are heard on expiration. Wheezing is caused by the collapse of airways. During expiration, the positive pressure outside the alveoli tends to collapse the small air passages, causing wheezing sounds.

4. **d** nonproductive cough

Rationale

During an asthma attack, D. will be encouraged to cough in an effort to raise the mucus that is contributing to airway obstruction. However, during an attack, airway resistance increases, reducing his ability to cough effectively. His inability to move the mucus out of the obstructed airways makes him more dyspneic and cyanotic. Both are signs of respiratory compromise, suggesting ventilatory failure if not corrected. D.'s blood gases reveal a low oxygen level suggestive of hypoxia.

5. **b** dilate the bronchioles

Rationale

Aminophylline is a sympathomimetic agent that produces bronchodilatation and an increased mucociliary transport action in an attempt to open obstructed airways. Aminophylline stimulates the β-adrenergic receptors, thus increasing cyclic adenosine monophosphate (cAMP) and acting to inhibit release of mediator factors.

6. **c** viral or bacterial infection

Rationale

D. was exposed to an upper respiratory infection through his brother. An elevated white blood cell count is most likely a reaction to an infectious agent's entering the body. D. has no history of allergies at this time. Physical activity can precipitate asthma attacks but will not produce elevated white blood cell counts.

1. **c**   urolithiasis

Rationale

Urolithiasis is most consistent with the overall findings. Presence of blood and calcium oxalate crystals is highly indicative of urinary tract calculi when associated with Mr. G.'s clinical findings of flank and abdominal pain, vomiting, and week-long history of back discomfort. Pyelonephritis would most likely present with a urine containing white blood cell casts and increased bacteria. A complete blood count would probably reveal more significant leukocytosis, and the individual would probably be more ill-appearing and have less pain than Mr. G. Cystitis is not usually accompanied by calcium oxalate crystals, and urinalysis would reveal more bacteria with a normal hematologic white count. Nephrotic syndrome presents with massive proteinuria, edema, hyperlipidemia, and hypoalbuminemia, none of which reflect this individual's clinical findings. Absence of rebound tenderness and relatively low white cell count without stab cells make appendicitis less likely.

2. **e**   hyperparathyroidism

Rationale

The portrait of a renal calculus former includes the following characteristics: male, age 10 to 55, Caucasian; living in the Southeast or Southwest United States (the "Stone Belt"); diet high in purines, calcium, or oxalates; family history of kidney stones; sedentary life-style; presence of hyperparathyroidsm or gout. All of these factors increase a person's risk for developing calculi. Mr. G.'s calcium and urate results were normal, excluding the likelihood of hyperparathyroidism or gout. Although there is no medical documentation, the intermittent hematuria his father and grandfather experienced suggests calculi. Individuals whose relatives are stone formers have a 10 times higher incidence of renal lithiasis. The overall incidence of renal calculi in the United States is 1 in 1000. In the Stone Belt regions, however, 15 of every 1000 hospital admissions are related to calculi. This finding may be correlated with high environmental temperature resulting in increased fluid loss and urine concentration.

3. **d** intravenous pyelography

Rationale

Many diagnosticians feel that an intravenous pyelogram (IVP) should be performed as quickly as possible to evaluate the presence of renal calculi, especially if they are nonradiopaque (uric acid, cystine). This roentgenogram study can localize the position of the stone(s), as well as provide vital information about the structure and function of the entire renal system. Cystoscopy can evaluate only visible lesions in the urethra and bladder. Renal calculi frequently are trapped in ureters or the pelvocaliceal systems. Retrograde pyelography is far riskier than IVP and is utilized more often as a last attempt to visualize kidney structures in individuals with decreased renal function. Angiography would only provide information about renal blood flow, not stone location per se. Abdominal ultrasound is not specific enough, though it might be used for persons who are allergic to IVP dye. A plain abdominal film (KUB) would probably be equally useful (and less expensive), though only radiopaque calculi could be seen.

4. **d** The individual should be taught to measure his urine pH and increase fluids

Rationale

Many calculi pass spontaneously. Until recently those that did not were surgically removed. A lithotripter is a machine, developed in Germany, that can pulverize kidney stones with shock waves sent through a tub of water. This could prevent costly and painful surgery for many sufferers. Treatment would cost $2000 less than the average expense of surgically removing kidney stones. It is important, regardless of the treatment for stone removal, to obtain the stones and analyze their contents. This analysis is essential in developing future plans to prevent recurrence. A person at home or in the hospital must strain the urine and save any gravel obtained. Urine strainers can be purchased; nylon stockings or gauze is equally effective and economical. Many stones are pH-sensitive. Individuals are taught to monitor their urine pH and adjust their diet accordingly. Increased fluids and activity are important in preventing not only urinary calculi but other urologic disorders. Renal calculi usually present with severe pain. Initially individuals require narcotic anagesics such as morphine or meperidine to relieve their pain.

5. **b** acid

Rationale

Calcium oxalate crystals are most frequently found in alkaline urine. It would be best for this individual to remain in a more acid range.

6. **e**   more than one of the above

Rationale

A staghorn calculus is often large and has many fingerlike projections into the surrounding kidney tissue. They often grow to enormous size and can actually fill an entire kidney. They may be relatively asymptomatic while they silently rob the kidney of its function. Until recently open surgical removal of the stone (pyelolithotomy) or of the entire kidney (nephrectomy) was the only treatment option. With the advent of the lithotripter, such stones may be treated by shock wave therapy and may be able to pass without surgical intervention. In the case of a very large, partially obstructing staghorn stone, a percutaneous catheter is placed into the kidney and the stone is bombarded by ultrasonic disruption. The PCNL tube functions as an alternative pathway for stone fragment exit. Unlike open surgery, these procedures do not incapacitate the individual for months, and once the PCNL tube is removed (a simple radiological procedure), the individual is left with a tiny scar where the tube was inserted. Ureterolithotomy would not be possible for a stone embedded in the body of the kidney. Only ureteral stones may be treated in this manner.

7. **a**   obstruction

Rationale

Obstruction is a predisposing factor in the development of urinary tract infections and chronic pyelonephritis. Depending on the location and severity of the obstruction, irreversible destruction of renal structures and diminution of function would result. Pain, hematuria, and crystalluria are frequently associated with renal calculi but in and of themselves are less potentially damaging than obstruction.

8. **c**   increased water; decreased spinach, asparagus, oranges

Rationale

To prevent further calcium oxalate stone formation, Mr. G. must attempt to increase hydration and avoid foods that are high in oxalate (spinach, rhubarb, asparagus, parsley, garlic, tomatoes, oranges, fruit juices, tea, cocoa [Ovaltine]) or calcium (dairy products). His fluid intake should be approximately 3 to 4 quarts a day, preferably water. If uric acid stones were present, intake of chicken, pork, beef, salmon, and mutton should be curtailed, since these foods contain moderate quantities of purine precursors. Unfortunately renal lithiasis formation is such a complex, multifactorial process that simply altering dietary intake will not guarantee prevention of kidney stones.

1. **d**   lack of renal perfusion

   Rationale
   GFR is dependent on renal blood flow, that is, an intact cardiovascular system. Mrs. S.'s massive bleeding resulted in hypovolemia, hypotension, and shock. Hypovolemia leads to decreased renal blood flow, which in turn causes decreased filtration pressure in the glomerulus. Because glomerular filtration (and production of urine) is driven partly by the pressure exerted from renal blood flow, anything that compromises renal blood flow can result in decreased urine output.

2. **c**   causing generalized vasoconstriction, increasing sodium and water resorption in the renal tubules, and concentrating the urine

   Rationale
   Renin release results in generalized vasoconstriction, elevating the blood pressure in an attempt to maintain an adequate circulation. ADH acts to increase circulatory volume by causing water reabsorption in the distal renal tubules and collecting ducts. Aldosterone is a mineralocorticoid produced in the adrenal gland as a result of stimulation of the renin-angiotensin system. In Mrs. S.'s case, decreased renal blood flow stimulated renin release from the kidneys, which then triggered the production of angiotensins I, II, and III. Angiotensin then stimulated the release of aldosterone. Aldosterone works in Henle's loop, distal convoluted tubule, and collecting ducts to increase reabsorption of sodium. Since water follows sodium, the body also reabsorbs more water from the kidneys, thus increasing circulatory blood volume.

3. **c**   orthostatic changes in vital signs, edema, weight, and lung sounds

Rationale

Mrs. S.'s fluid status can be assessed, in part, by evaluating cardiovascular function. If she were hypovolemic, one might see a drop in blood pressure and an increased pulse rate when she moved from lying to standing (orthostatic changes). Fluid overload (hypervolemia) might be manifested as weight gain, edema, jugular venous distention, or pulmonary congestion (lung crackles). Normally urine output, specific gravity, and electrolytes can be used as indicators of fluid status, but in Mrs. S.'s case, they are not very useful. This is because the tubular cell damage has made the kidneys unable to retain sodium or to control the concentration of the urine. The urine specific gravity becomes fixed at plasma levels (1.010) and the urine sodium levels are high. These measures are no longer accurate indicators of fluid status in Mrs. S.

4. **b**   contributing to tubular necrosis by increasing ischemia

Rationale

The tubular damage has caused a decrease in sodium resorption. The low sodium content in the distal tubule, along with decreased renal perfusion and continued sympathetic stimulation, stimulates the renin mechanism. The resulting generalized vasoconstriction constricts the renal blood vessels and decreases the GFR even more. That, in turn, contributes to cellular ischemia, setting up a vicious cycle increasing tubular necrosis.

5. **a**   electrocardiogram changes, weakness, dyspnea, irritability, and nausea

Rationale

Many of the symptoms of hyperkalemia are related to changes in cell membrane excitability caused by an increase in extracellular potassium. Mrs. S.'s blood pH is 7.20, indicating acidosis. In states of acidosis hydrogen ions enter the cell in exchange for potassium and sodium ions. These potassium ions enter the extracellular fluid and exert their effects on cell membranes. High levels of potassium cause the resting membrane potential to approach the threshold potential. This means the cell repolarizes more rapidly and is more irritable. This condition is reflected in tall, narrow T waves and shortened Q-T intervals on an electrocardiogram. With severe hyperkalemia this resting membrane potential can equal the threshold potential, thus preventing the cell from repolarizing at all. The electrocardiogram changes seen with severe hyperkalemia include depressed S-T segments, increased P-R intervals, and wider QRS complexes. Conduction slows (bradycardia) and eventually stops, leading to cardiac arrest. An unrepolarized cell cannot respond to a stimulus. If the cells in question are cardiac cells, cardiac standstill can be a natural consequence of hyperkalemia.

The muscle weakness and dyspnea can be explained in the same way. In addition, early neuromuscular irritability can lead to restlessness and gastrointestinal disturbances such as nausea, cramping, and diarrhea.

6. **a**   increased respiratory excretion of carbon dioxide (Kussmaul's respiration) and the blood buffer $NaHCO_3$

Rationale

Metabolic acidosis occurs when the hydrogen ion concentration increases or when the blood level of bicarbonate decreases. This state is reflected in lower blood pH and bicarbonate levels. The body has several buffer systems that act to compensate for these pH changes. The lungs act to rid the body of carbon dioxide by increasing the number and depth of respirations (Kussmaul's respirations). The excreted carbon dioxide is one product of the breakdown of carbonic acid; a major source of hydrogen ions in the blood. The other product is water. This form of compensation is activated early by the body.

Bicarbonate-carbonic acid buffering is another major compensatory factor. Normal bicarbonate levels are about 24 mEq/L in a 20:1 ratio with carbonic acid. A balance exists between the acids and bases when the ratio is maintained and pH is stable. The kidneys control the bicarbonate by reabsorbing it from the urine or by generating it from carbon dioxide and water. In Mrs. S.'s case, her kidneys are unable to maintain a bicarbonate balance, even though her lungs are decreasing the carbonic acid by blowing off carbon dioxide. In addition, normal kidneys also excrete hydrogen ions. For Mrs. S. this represents another compromised compensatory mechanism.

7. **b**   hypovolemia and hypokalemia

Rationale

Mrs. S. is in the diuretic phase of ATN, and, although her function continues to improve, her tubules are far from normal. Mrs. S.'s renal tubules are still unable to conserve fluid and electrolytes, as they wash out in the high urine output she is currently experiencing. Hypokalemia is just as deadly as hyperkalemia, and dehydration can lead to shock (though more slowly) just as massive blood loss can.

1. **d** all of the above

Rationale

Diabetes mellitus is a major cause of renal morbidity and mortality. Chronic renal disease accounts for 20% of deaths in diabetic persons under the age of 40. The term *diabetic neuropathy* is appied to the host of lesions that occur concurrently in the diabetic kidney. The most common lesions involve the glomeruli; however, diabetes also affects the arterioles, causing arteriolar sclerosis; predisposes to pylonephritis; and causes a variety of tubular lesions.

The morphologic changes in the glomeruli include (1) capillary basement membrane thickening, (2) diffuse diabetic glomerulosclerosis, and (3) nodular glomerulosclerosis. Diffuse glomerulosclerosis consists of diffuse increase in the mesangial matrix with proliferation of mesangial cells. This process is always associated with the overall thickening of the glomerular basement membrane. As the disease progresses, the mesangial area expands and obliterates the mesangial cells, eventually filling the entire glomerulus. These changes are not pathognomonic of diabetes and may resemble some stages of glomerulonephritis.

Nodular glomerosclerosis is also known as *intercapillary glomerulosclerosis*, or *Kimmelstiel-Wilson disease*. The lesions take the form of spherical hyaline masses situated in the periphery of the glomerulus. The nodules contain lipids and fibrin and, often, trapped mesangial cells. Eventually, the entire glomerulus is converted to a hyaline sclerotic mass. This type of nodular lesion is virtually pathognomonic of diabetes.

The pathogenesis of diabetic glomerulosclerosis is closely linked to the pathogenesis of the generalized microangiopathy occurring in diabetes. Much evidence suggests that diabetic microangiopathy is caused by the metabolic defect (i.e., the insulin deficiency or the resultant hyperglycemia). The exact mechanism for the initiation or modulation of diabetic glomerulosclerosis is still unknown. One recently investigated theory involves the hyperfiltration that is known to occur in the diabetic state. Experimental evidence indicates that the contractile ability of the mesangial cells is reduced by hyperglycemia or the insulin-deficient state. This could result in glomerular vasodilatation and increased interglomerular plasma flow, filtration pressure, and hyperfiltration. It is possible that the glomerular changes are actually caused by these hemodynamic alterations. Whether precise control of blood glucose in diabetes prevents glomerulopathy remains an important but unanswered question.

2. **b**   loss of bicarbonate in the urine

Rationale

The body, through normal metabolism of an average diet, produces an acid residue of 50 to 100 mEq/day. In renal failure, particularly chronic renal failure, all three of the kidney's mechanisms for excreting acid and preserving bicarbonate are impaired, resulting in varying degrees of metabolic acidosis. Acidosis may not be noted, however, until glomerular filtration is reduced to one quarter or less of normal.

This metabolic acidosis may be a hyperchloremic acidosis caused by failure of ammonia production, reabsorption of bicarbonate, or both. With failure of complete reabsorption of bicarbonate, sodium is lost in the urine. This reduces the concentration of bicarbonate in the renal absorbate and in body fluids. Since sodium and chloride are ingested in almost equivalent amounts, the loss of sodium combined with bicarbonate in the urine leads to relative hyperchloremia. Excretion of sodium bicarbonate results in an increase in the chloride concentration of the extracellular fluid equivalent to the fall in bicarbonate. Since the urine in this situation is relatively alkaline, little sodium can be conserved by renal production of ammonium.

Sulfuric acids and other organic acids are produced during normal metabolism, particularly of amino acids. The anions of these acids are largely excreted but poorly absorbed once filtered. Beause of the inadequate ammonia production, they cannot be excreted as their ammonium salts; instead obligate excretion of fixed cation, generally sodium, occurs. Thus H_2SO_4 is formed in the body, but $HaSO_4$ is excreted. The retained hydrogen ions cause acidosis. This more often occurs in earlier stages of renal failure.

With more advanced renal failure about one half of individuals are unable to reabsorb all the filtered bicarbonate. Wastage of bicarbonate and metabolic acidosis occur. The other half of individuals with chronic renal failure who are not bicarbonate wasters still become acidotic because ammonia production is not augmented enough to meet the needs of hydrogen ion excretion, even when urine acidification is maximal.

With advancing renal disease and declining glomerular filtration rates, hyperchloremia recedes as other anions, such as sulfate, phosphate, and urea, are retained. These anions gradually displace chloride. It should be noted, however, that it is the failure to excrete the hydrogen ion of sulfuric and phosphoric acids, not the retention of their ions, that causes the acidosis of renal failure.

It should be apparent that the exact mechanism for creating the acidotic state varies considerably with the degree of renal compromise. It should also be noted that there is much yet unknown about renal physiology and no matter what phase of renal physiology is being discussed, the principles believed to be true may now be modified by further knowledge.

3. **d**   all of the above

Rationale

Anemia is extremely common in advanced stages of renal failure. A roughly inverse correlation has been found between the blood urea nitrogen concentration and the hemoglobin level. This is illustrated by Mr. B.'s high blood urea nitrogen of 88 mg/dl and his low hemoglobin of 11 g.

Bleeding tendencies, also common in chronic renal failure, may contribute to the anemia. They are manifested by frequent nose bleeds, gastrointestinal bleeding, bruising, and so on. Thrombocytopenia may be a cause of bleeding but most likely is a problem related to the quality of the platelets rather than quantity.

As a general rule the anemia is normochromic and normocytic. The number of circulating reticulocytes in the peripheral blood is low or normal, and the bone marrow is hypoplastic, indicating a general depression of the red cell series. The cause of the bone marrow suppression is not known. Presumably there are circulating factors that appear to inhibit the bone marrow response to erythropoietin, a peptide hormone that generally stimulates red cell production. This substance is produced chiefly in the kidneys.

In addition to the reduced response of the bone marrow to erythropoietin, there is a reduced secretion of erythropoietin by the diseased kidneys. Deficiency of this hormone undoubtedly contributes significantly to the anemia.

Although reduced erythrocyte production is probably the major cause of anemia, the increased rate of destruction of red blood cells is also a significant factor. The red cells of the uremic person are abnormally fragile. Substances in the uremic plasma, as yet unidentified, reversibly inhibit red cell membrane sodium potassium adenosinetriphosphatase (Na,K-ATPase) and cause increased erythrocyte fragility. Because of the increased fragility the cell life is shortened in general and is probably more susceptible to trauma induced by dialysis and ultrafiltration.

4. **e**   a and b only

Rationale

The kidney contributes to the control of blood pressure through several mechanisms. Derangements in these mechanisms may contribute to the development of hypertension. These mechanisms can be grouped into two categories: (1) those involved in the maintenance of extracellular fluid volume and (2) those involved with the secretion of neurohumoral messengers by the kidneys. The kidneys may form increased amounts of vasoactive substances. The renin-angiotensin-aldosterone axis is activated by (1) decreased afferent arteriolar pressure, (2) decreased sodium or chloride load in the macula densa, and (3) epinephrine and direct neurostimulation.

The enzyme renin is formed and stored in the juxtaglomerular cells of the kidney, from which it is released into renal venous blood. It acts on the plasma substance angiotensinogen, converting it to angiotensin I. This substance is further converted within the circulation to angiotensin II by a converting enzyme. Angiotensin II is a powerful vasoconstrictor that alone can cause a dramatic increase in blood pressure. In addition angiotensin II stimulates the adrenal cortex to secrete aldosterone. Under normal conditions any increased renin secretion is quickly corrected by a negative feedback mechanism, but in renal failure the feedback control mechanisms are altered. In about 10% of individuals with chronic renal failure, renin hypertension appears to be the predominant cause of hypertension.

The remaining 90% of individuals with renal failure have hypertension resulting from volume overload. The kidney is the primary organ controlling the sodium content of body fluids. Diseased kidneys are not able to adjust sodium content, thus leading to overexpansion of the extracellular fluid volume. This overexpansion leads to the large amount of edema commonly found in individuals with chronic renal failure, including Mr. B., as noted by the 3+ pitting edema in his lower extremities. This is enhanced by the fact that persons with renal failure also lose much protein, especially albumin, in their urine, leading to hypoproteinemia and hypoalbuminemia. Overexpansion of the extracellular fluid volume eventually leads to overexpansion of the intravascular volume. The relationship between excess intravascular volume and hypertension can be readily seen when one realizes that the determinants of cardiac output are heart rate and volume of venous return. The amount of venous return is very dependent on intravascular volume. Thus this increased intravascular fluid volume is a major cause of hypertension in individuals with renal failure.

Saying that hypertension results from either activation of the renin-angiotensin system or volume overload is a gross oversimplification. In actual fact each occurs to some extent in most cases of hypertension. There are other factors that contribute, in varying degrees, to the hypertensive state. One is the relative decrease in secretion of prostaglandins by the diseased kidneys. Prostaglandins are antihypertensive substances produced and secreted by normal kidneys. Loss of these substances may contribute to hypertension as well.

5. c decreasing glomerular filtration rate

Rationale
Creatinine is a substance released by muscle tissue and excreted through glomerular filtration in the kidneys. If the glomerular filtration rate (GFR) falls, as it does in renal failure, the blood level of creatinine rises. Thus plasma creatinine is an index of renal function. Mr. B.'s creatinine level of 8.1 mg/dl is quite high. His renal function is obviously impaired.

6. a Urinary concentration has become fixed at plasma levels as a result of severe renal failure

Rationale
The concentration of urine is also a function of glomerular filtration, in conjunction with circulating levels of antidiuretic hormone (ADH). As the GFR falls, the kidneys begin to lose their ability to dilute or concentrate urine. When GFR reaches 15% to 20% of normal and nephron and tubule damage is very severe, the concentration of urine is fixed at the osmolality of plasma, about 1.010. Mr. B.'s specific gravity of 1.009 is undoubtedly a reflection of his progressive renal failure.

1. **d** sympathetic nervous system mediated reflex

Rationale
Postoperative individuals have been shown to have increases in the blood plasma and bowel levels of adrenaline and noradrenaline. These findings have led to the current hypothesis that the sympathetic nervous system inhibits normal bowel motility. The increased levels of adrenaline may be related to either or both the actual surgery and manipulation of the bowel at the time of surgery. Opiates such as morphine have also been implicated in the duration of the ileus. However, these studies are conflicting in their findings.

2. **c** duration of surgery

Rationale
The duration of surgery has not been positively linked with the duration of ileus. Ileus has occurred even after minor surgical procedures. Neither has a correlation between ileus and extent of bowel manipulation been established. Hypokalemia can lead to bowel hypotonia, necessitating postoperative correction of electrolyte imbalances. Peritonitis has a toxic and metabolically disturbing effect, thus increasing sympathetic and hypotonic effects. Retroperitoneal tissue aggravation results in reflex stimulation of the sympathetic outflow and thus increases sympathetic effects.

3. **d** alkalosis (metabolic) and respiratory acidosis

Rationale
Both postoperative vomiting and lost gastric secretions lead to electrolyte disturbances. This disturbance is caused by the direct electrolytes lost with these secretions. Metabolic alkalosis produced by acid loss will ensue if treatment is not initiated. Compensatory mechanisms will result in respiratory acidosis if metabolic alkalosis is left unchecked.

4. **c**   flatus and/or stool passed

Rationale

Radiological and auscultative studies have shown that in the absence of complications, contractions of the small intestines return within a few hours of *routine* laparotomy. By contrast the large bowel remains quiescent for 1 or 2 days. The absence of bowel sounds is indicative of an empty small bowel. Introduction of air and/or fluid into the stomach produces bowel sounds as it passes through the small bowel. Thus postoperative distention is usually gas trapped in the atonic colon. Passage of flatus and/or stool is the best indicator of returning colonic motility.

5. **d**   hypertension

Rationale

Resumption of diet when colonic activity has not fully resumed can further increase distension, thereby diminishing effectiveness of already sluggish peristalsis. Electrolyte imbalances, as already discussed, can lead to bowel hypotonia, as can diabetes.

6. **a**   abdominal film demonstrating a local loop of dilated small bowel in the absence of gas in the colon

Rationale

The typical clinical features of ileus are abdominal distention, nausea and vomiting, or large nasogastric output and no flatus or stool. If distension is significant, tachypnea resulting from elevated hemidiaphragms and tachycardia (mild) caused by pain and anxiety can ensue. The absence of gas in the large bowel, in view of the preceding, is indicative of intestinal obstruction. Accurate diagnosis is essential in differentiating obstruction from ileus as treatment modalities differ. Conservative therapy, such as oral intake restriction, gastric decompression, and fluid and electrolyte management, is indicated for ileus. Laparotomy, which aggravates ileus, is the urgent treatment for obstruction.

7. **a**   enemas/cathartics

Rationale

Gastric decompression prevents further colonic distention with air or fluid. Analgesics are useful in treating pain and anxiety, which when left untreated can result in the individual's swallowing air, which further dilates the colon. Enemas/cathartics are not used primarily because they can be detrimental in cases of misdiagnosed obstruction. Often enemas only increase the amount of fluid already harbored by the atonic colon.

1. **d**   all of the above

   Rationale
   Research evidence suggests that smoking is positively linked to ulcer formation. However, the physiology of this link is not clearly understood. Anti-inflammatory agents (aspirin, prednisone, etc.) decrease mucosal resistance by inhibiting mucous synthesis and causing abnormal permeability. In terms of hereditary factors, an increased incidence of ulcers has been observed among parents and siblings of individuals with ulcers when compared to the general population. It has been hypothesized that people genetically predisposed to ulcer formation who become stressed are more likely to develop ulcers.

2. **b**   increased back-diffusion of ingested acid into the mucosa

   Rationale
   The major contributing factor is hypersecretion of acid in individuals with a duodenal ulcer, which causes a greater mass of parietal cells than found in normal persons. Individuals with duodenal ulcers are abnormally sensitive to gastrin and have increased submaximal secretion. Also, rapid emptying of the stomach diminishes the buffering effects of a meal and compromises the buffering reserve provided by pancreatic bicarbonate secretions. Gastric ulceration is believed to be primarily related to a break in the "mucosal barrier." This barrier allows secretion of hydrochloric acid into the stomach without injuring epithelial cells. Damage to the mucosal barrier, conceivably by reflux of bile acids into the stomach, allows back-diffusion of hydrogen ions, causing mucosal inflammation.

3. **h**   a, b, d

Rationale

Three common major complications of peptic ulcer disease are gastric outlet obstruction, hemorrhage, and perforation. Hemorrhage is the most common complication; it occurs more often with gastric ulcers because they may penetrate into an artery. Bleeding may be manifested as either hematemesis (blood in vomitus) or melena (blood in stools). Acute exacerbation is usually accompanied by bleeding, accentuated pain, nausea, and vomiting. Symptoms ultimately depend on the severity of the hemorrhage and resulting occurrence of hypovolemic shock. Intervention is focused on treating the hypovolemic shock, preventing dehydration and electrolyte imbalance, stopping the bleeding, and providing rest. Symptomatic relief is achieved by placing a nasogastric tube into the stomach. The rationale is to keep the stomach empty and reduce stimulus for hydrochloric acid and pepsin secretion. If symptoms do not respond to conservative treatment, especially if perforation is considered a possibility, surgical intervention is indicated.

4. **a**   dumping syndrome

Rationale

The dumping syndrome is a postprandial problem, occuring more often in men than women and usually appearing 1 to 3 weeks after surgery when the individual attempts to consume larger meals. The symptoms, as noted in the case description, may occur while the person is eating or 15 to 30 minutes after eating; symptoms usually disappear within the hour.

With the storage capacity of the stomach decreased by surgery, food enters the small intestine in larger quantities and at a faster rate. This hypertonic bolus of food draws extracellular fluid into the lumen of the bowel, thereby decreasing plasma volume. The signs and symptoms may result from abdominal distention within the small intestine, drop in circulating plasma volume, or decrease in cardiac output. The decrease in plasma volume accounts for additional signs and symptoms, which include palpitations, tachycardia, syncope, and decreased blood pressure.

The syndrome usually lasts from a few days to several weeks. Few individuals require surgery to relieve these symptoms. Ms. K. should have six small feedings a day. Meals should contain foods reduced in carbohydrates, restricted in refined sugars, and moderate in fat and protein. Fat and protein tend to leave the stomach more slowly and do not draw fluid into the intestine. Fluids should be consumed between meals and not with meals.

5. **b**   afferent loop obstruction

Rationale

An afferent loop obstruction may occur as a result of a Billroth II surgical procedure. Surgical intervention requires removal of the affected stomach area and anastomosis of the remaining stomach to the jejunum. An afferent loop of the duodeum is created. Hernia, stenosis, or adhesions in the surgical area may cause partial obstruction. Obstruction delays stomach emptying, causing symptoms of fullness and pain.

1. **b**   ascites and edema

Rationale

Ascites is the accumulation of large volumes of fluids within the peritoneal cavity. It occurs often in alcoholic cirrhosis as well as other types of liver disease. Related complications include edema and decreased urine volume. Together these result in fluid and electrolyte imbalances and derangements in protein metabolism in the individual with liver disease. Ascites can be detected when approximately 500 ml of fluid has accumulated in the peritoneal cavity. Fluid and solutes pass across the vascular membrane as a result of the following mechanisms:

Decreased plasma colloid oncotic pressure: Albumin is low in cirrhotic individuals as a result of expanded plasma volume, impaired synthesis in the liver, and loss of albumin into the peritoneal cavity. This hypoalbuminemia reduces plasma oncotic pressure as the total plasma protein concentration is decreased and water is lost to the extravascular space.

Hyperaldosteronism: This is a secondary condition common in cirrhotic persons with ascites. The excessive sodium reabsorption in the distal tubule of the kidney further compounds water retention, resulting in increased plasma volume. The increased aldosterone secretion occurs as a result of a reduction in renal blood flow and impaired metabolism and excretion of aldosterone by the liver.

Impaired water excretion: Renal excretion of water is impaired as a result of decreased renal blood flow and, in some cases, high levels of circulating antidiuretic hormone.

Management of ascites is usually accomplished by strict sodium and water restriction and diuretic therapy. A life-threatening complication of ascites is respiratory depression caused by excessive fluid's limiting the expansion of the diaphragm. This may necessitate paracentesis to remove fluid and decrease respiratory embarrassment.

2. **a**   esophageal varices

Rationale

Alcohol acts with a dose-related toxic effect on the liver and disrupts liver metabolism. Chronic alcohol abuse results in destruction of hepatic tissue, fibrosis, and permanent cell damage. Formation of fibrotic nodules blocks normal blood flow. As this obstruction occurs, pressure in the portal vein increases. Collateral circulation develops to shunt blood back to the right side of the heart in order to decrease the pressure in the portal vein. This portal hypertension eventually affects blood vessels supplying the portal system, including esophageal vessels, thus the formation of esophageal varices. Hemorrhage from these, if untreated or massive, can be fatal.

3. **c**   hepatic encephalopathy

Rationale

Hepatic (portal-systemic) encephalopathy is a complex brain syndrome that causes major disturbances of the central nervous system. It is caused by metabolic changes and may be acute or chronic. Four major elements are usually present in this syndrome, including (1) advanced liver disease with or without portal-systemic shunts, (2) disturbance in level of consciousness with a progression of confusion to stupor and coma, (3) shifting neurological signs, and (4) electroencephalogram changes. This physiological defect results from a shunting of portal blood directly into systemic circulation, bypassing the liver, and severe hepatocellular damage and dysfunction. The result of these is the presence of toxic substances that are absorbed from the intestine, bypassing liver metabolism. These toxic substances then accumulate in the brain.

Ammonia is a common toxin found in elevated levels in individuals with encephalopathy. Hyperammonemia occurs in conjunction with systemic alkalosis and gastrointestinal bleeding (nitrogenous substance in the colon). Treatment is aimed at reducing ammonia production in the colon, eliminating or treating any precipitating factors, and providing support of vital functions. Lactulose was given to reduce Mr. S.'s ammonia levels. Lactulose acidifies the colon, helping ammonia combine with hydrogen for excretion in the feces.

4. **b**   interruption of normal clotting mechanisms

Rationale

Blood clotting represents a series of enzymatic reactions involving a variety of plasma proteins, most of which are synthesized by the liver. Prothrombin, one of the most important, is a precursor to thrombin, a proteolytic enzyme. Thrombin acts to convert fibrinogen to fibrin but requires the presence of sufficient levels of vitamin K in the liver to accomplish this. In the presence of hepatocellular dysfunction these precursors do not occur normally; thus, the sequence of coagulation is disrupted. This is seen clinically by active bleeding and evidenced in lab studies showing increased PT and partial thromboplastin time (PTT) which measure adequacy of extrinsic system factors and presence of normal levels of intrinsic factors VIII and IX, respectively.

1. **c** The infant normally loses and replaces 25% of the total body water in 24 hours

   Rationale
   Infants have a very high rate of water turnover. They lose and replace 25% of their total body reservoir of water every 24 hours. In contrast adults turn over only 6%. Anything that interferes with fluid intake or increases body losses rapidly precipitates dehydration in this vulnerable population.

   Other factors that contribute to the infant's response to fluid alterations are higher metabolic rate and larger water content than the adult's. In a newborn 80% of the total body weight is water. The child has reached the adult water content of 60% total body weight by the age of 3. The infant also has an immature renal system that prevents concentration and retention of fluids.

2. **b** decreased peripheral perfusion

   Rationale
   When intravascular fluid or plasma is initially lost through diarrhea, the interstitial fluid shifts into the blood vessels in an attempt to maintain circulating blood volume. When fluid loss exceeds the body's ability to compensate, the circulating volume is diminished, vasoconstriction occurs in the peripheral vessels, and decreased perfusion of tissues is evidenced by weak peripheral pulses, delayed capillary filling, and mottled or grayish skin color.

3. **b**   The infectious agent invades the gastrointestinal mucosa and alters the balance of water and electrolytes

Rationale

Acute gastroenteritis is most often viral (70% to 80% of cases), though some are bacterial (10% to 20% of cases). These infectious agents cause diarrhea by altering the balance of fluid and electrolyte movement in the bowel.

Normally a large volume of fluid is processed by the bowel and 90% of fluid absorption takes place in the small intestine. This absorption is passive, as water follows electrolytes along an osmotic gradient. Fluid and electrolyte movement is also normally bidirectional, thus helping maintain a balance.

It is believed that the virus associated with gastroenteritis damages the villous epithelial cells, replacing them with immature crypt cells. This decreases the amount of absorptive area in the intestine. The virus also stimulates electrolyte secretion into the intestine. Water follows the osmotic gradient, causing watery stools. Though the mechanism in bacterial gastroenteritis is somewhat different, secretory diarrhea also results.

4. **b**   intravascular

Rationale

During the first phase of fluid replacement in dehydration, the goal is to replace the intravascular fluid volume that has been lost rapidly so that blood will carry oxygen and nutrients to body cells and remove waste products. It also enables the kidneys to function more efficiently. In isonatremic dehydration most of the water is lost through the extracellular space; the intravascular volume is one of the chief components of that space.

5. **d**   lactic acid production secondary to decreased perfusion

Rationale

The hydrogen ion disturbance seen most frequently with vomiting and diarrhea is metabolic acidosis. Several factors that contribute to this are (1) diminished perfusion of tissues, causing anaerobic metabolism and production of lactic acid and other acid metabolites; (2) decreased renal function preventing the kidneys from excreting hydrogen ions; (3) bicarbonate loss in diarrheal stools; and (4) lack of oral intake, causing catabolism of fats and proteins with production of organic acids.

6. **a**   acidosis

Rationale

Acidosis causes hydrogen ions to enter body cells in exchange for potassium ions that are released into the intravascular compartment. Impaired renal function also causes retention of potassium ions. Both events may result in high serum potassium levels when the individual may have had significant potassium losses in gastrointestinal secretions. To prevent complications of possible hyperkalemia, it is recommended that intravenous potassium be withheld until urine output is established. Potassium must then be given to replace losses.

7. **a** isonatremic

Rationale

K.L.'s sodium level is 136 mEq/L, which is within the normal range. This means she is losing water and electrolytes in a balanced way. Isonatremic dehydration is most common with acute gastroenteritis. Hyponatremic dehydration occurs when sodium losses are proportionately greater than water losses or when low-sodium, low-solute fluids are used to replace diarrheal fluids. Hypernatremic dehydration is the opposite in that more fluid than sodium is lost or high-sodium fluids are used as replacement. In oral fluid replacement, the cause of both hyponatremic and hypernatremic dehydration is often the use of homemade oral solutions containing too little or too much electrolyte.

1. **c**   secondary

   Rationale
   Mr. D. has secondary degenerative joint disease, most likely caused by the developmental epiphyseal ossification disorder he experienced at age 10. This disorder is the early calcification of the epiphyseal plate. Calcification normally occurs after puberty. Various sports that cause trauma in a joint have been associated with degenerative joint disease. Age is a primary etiologic factor in primary degenerative joint disease.

2. **a**   erosion of cartilage

   Rationale
   Loss of articular cartilage leaves the underlying bone unprotected; as a result the bone becomes sclerotic and cyst formation is common. Osteophyte formation is associated with cartilage loss but does not account for the cyst formation.

3. **c**   sclerosis of the femur and osteophytes

   Rationale
   The characteristic pathophysiological changes seen in degenerative joint disease are cartilage destruction, osteophyte formation, and sclerosis of the bone underlying the cartilage. Shortening of extremities is not characteristic of degenerative joint disease.

4. **b**   osteophyte and cyst formations

Rationale

The actual causes of pain in degenerative joint disease are poorly understood. Generally the joint pain is attributed to osteophyte formation, cyst formation, and stretching of the joint capsule. Cartilage itself lacks nerve fibers and is believed insensitive to pain. Free-floating cartilage fragments in the joint space may initiate inflammation that may contribute to the joint pain. A joint with limited range of motion will be painful when movement stretches the joint capsule.

5. **a**   damage to the joint's supporting structure

Rationale

Joint instability (giving way in a joint) is usually the result of damage to a joint's supporting structures (joint capsule, ligaments, tendons). Chronic inflammation may initiate or aggravate degenerative changes, potentially rendering a joint unstable. Neurological disorders associated with loss of pain or proprioceptive reflexes may contribute to joint instability, but there is no evidence of a neurological disorder in Mr. D.'s case.

6. **d**   degeneration of articular cartilage

Rationale

Degeneration of articular cartilage is responsible for the limited range of motion in a joint; the degree of limitation depends on the extent of cartilage degeneration. Loss of proprioceptive reflexes in a joint is usually associated with hypermobility rather than limitation of movement.

1. **d**   articular cartilage destruction

   Rationale

   The loss of articular cartilage accounts for the loss of movement function in the hip joint. Without articular cartilage friction between the opposing bony surfaces is increased, making movement in the joint difficult. Pannus formation may be one of the factors responsible for cartilage destruction, but evidence does not support the conclusion that pannus formation itself limits joint mobility. Evidence of joint rupture is lacking in Mrs. O.'s case. Synovial edema may account for limited range of motion in early rheumatoid arthritis. However, given the lengthy history of rheumatoid arthritis and the loss of articular cartilage, very little synovial membrane probably persists in the left hip.

2. **c**   systemic nature of the disease

   Rationale

   Rheumatoid arthritis is a systemic autoimmune disease that affects connective tissue throughout the body. Although exposure to viruses has been shown to stimulate the production of rheumatoid factor, the presence of rheumatoid factor alone does not cause rheumatoid arthritis. The same is true of IgG: its presence is not responsible for rheumatoid arthritis.

3. **b**   lysosomal degradation

   Rationale

   Lysosomal enzymes produced by leukocytes are believed responsible for the destruction of articular cartilage in rheumatoid arthritis. The enzymes break down the collagen fibers and the protein polysaccharides of articular cartilage. Immune complexes initiate the inflammatory process that attracts leukocytes to the cartilage. Antigen-antibody formation results in the production of rheumatoid factors that combine with IgG to form immune complexes.

4. **a** preventing decreased activity, which can result in muscle atrophy

   Rationale
   Joint deformities lead to physical limitations. This limiting is compounded by pain experienced by Mrs. O. when she tries to move. Atrophy of the muscles around involved joints quickly follows limited motion. Range of motion exercises will help improve function, as well as strengthen involved musculature.

5. **c** formation of cysts

   Rationale
   Formation of cysts is a complication of rheumatoid arthritis. Cysts are the result of an excessive buildup of inflammatory exudate in synovial cavities. These cysts may rupture, causing additional inflammation in nearby tissue.

6. **a** to combat the inflammatory response activated by immune complexes

   Rationale
   Steroids are anti-inflammatory agents used to treat the inflammatory response that is activated by rheumatoid arthritis by the immune complexes. The inflammatory response includes activation of lymphocytes and the complement and kinin systems.

1. **a**   hypovolemic shock

   Rationale
   Burn shock is caused by a massive shift of fluids out of the blood vessels. As the capillaries become more permeable to water, sodium, and proteins, there is a shift into the interstitial spaces from the intravascular spaces. This decreases the blood volume, diminishing cardiac output.

2. **b**   facial edema

   Rationale
   Loss of capillary seal in burn shock results in generalized edema affecting all areas of the body, not just the burned tissue. This edema leads to mechanical obstruction of the upper airway. Early nasal intubation is the treatment of choice. The oral and nasal pharynx are efficient heat exchangers, and direct thermal insult to the lower respiratory tract is rare.

3. **b**   leakage of intracellular fluids from the capillaries

   Rationale
   As a result of leakage of intravascular fluid, plasma, sodium, potassium, and albumin to extravascular spaces (loss of capillary seal), the intravascular fluid becomes viscous, leading to increased hematocrit.

4. **d**   restoring adequate blood supply to the distal areas

   Rationale
   Circulation to extremities may be severely impaired by circumferential burns in combination with edema formation. This edema plus the decreased elasticity of the burn area may act as a tourniquet, necessitating escharotomies to restore circulation to compromised extremities.

5. **a**   in third-degree burns the dermis has been destroyed

Rationale

In third-degree burns both the epidermis and the dermis are destroyed. The dermis houses such structures as nerve endings, sebaceous glands, and hair follicles. In second-degree burns the exposed nerve endings are stimulated and signals are transmitted by the efferent fibers of the sensory system.

6. **b**   Ringer's lactate closely resembles extracellular fluid in composition and helps rapidly replace the fluid being lost from the extracellular compartments

Rationale

Initial fluid resuscitation is critical to all individuals who have suffered more than a 40% TBSA. The goal of fluid replacement is to stabilize the cardiac output. Ringer's lactate is the fluid of choice because it most normally resembles the physiological composition of the extracellular fluid being lost. The amount that is given depends on the weight of the individual as well as the percentage of the TBSA. Usually within a 24-hour period the cells are able to seal themselves off adequately so that cellular integrity is restored. Ringer's lactate has no effect on the plasma volume level, and this loss will have to be treated with plasma infusion.

7. **c**   The sodium loss resulting from the hydrotherapy must be minimized as much as possible

Rationale

Bath water is hypotonic and tends to draw vital sodium from the cell. To minimize this loss, hydrotherapy time is calculated around maximizing effectiveness while minimizing disadvantages. Hydrotherapy is useful for removing topical agents, such as the antibiotics (Bacitracin and Sulfamylon Acetate Cream) used on Mr. B., and for softening the eschar formation to increase comfort and range of motion.

8. **d**   He is beginning to present with signs of hypovolemic shock

Rationale

Abdominal distention and/or paralytic ileus tends to develop in the majority of persons who experience a greater than 20% TBSA the first 24 hours after the burn trauma. This phenomenon is most likely related to the "fight-or-flight" response to stress. Intestinal peristaltic action decreases as the body prepares to deal with the stressors at hand. Treatment for this symptom is insertion of a nasogastric tube until the bowel demonstrates signs of more normal functioning.

9. **a**   A gentle constant pressure should be applied to the newly grafted areas for approximately 1 year to promote circulation

Rationale

The low counterpressure that is provided by the application of the Jobst stockings helps to control hypertrophic scarring successfully as well as to reduce the edema around the graft sites.

Index

Acquired immune deficiency syndrome (AIDS), 9, 119
Acute lymphocytic leukemia (ALL), 44, 150
Acute renal failure, 85, 182
Alcoholic cirrhosis, 97, 193
Alzheimer-type senile dementia, 20, 126
Anemia, iron deficiency, 41, 146
Arthritis, rheumatoid, 104, 200
Asthma, 79, 177
Bacterial meningitis, 29, 134
Breast cancer, 13, 121
Bronchopneumonia, 73, 173
Burns, 106, 202
Cancer, breast, 13, 121
Cardiomyopathy, 61, 164
Cerebral vascular accident (CVA), 26, 132
Chronic renal failure, 88, 185
Coagulation, disseminated intravascular, 47, 153
Congestive heart failure (CHF), 54, 159
Coranary artery occlusion, 58, 161
Cushing syndrome, 39, 144
Cystic fibrosis (CF), 76, 175
Degenerative joint disease, 102, 198
Dehydration, 99, 195
Dementia, senile, 20, 126
Diabetes mellitus (DM), 36, 141
Disseminated intravascular coagulation (DIC), 47, 153

Down syndrome, 3, 113
Emphysema, 70, 171
Gastroenteritis, 99, 195
Graves disease, 33, 138
Hemophilia A, 50, 155
Hypertension, 54, 159
Hyperthyroidism, 33, 138
Hypovolemic shock, 64, 167
Ileus, surgical, 91, 189
Iron deficiency anemia, 41, 146
Leukemia, acute lymphocytic, 44, 150
Lung cancer, 17, 124
Meningitis, bacterial, 29, 134
Myocardial infarction (MI), 58, 161
Peptic ulcer disease, 94, 191
Rheumatoid arthritis, 104, 200
Senile dementia of the Alzheimer type (SDAT), 20, 126
Septicemia, 47, 153
Shock, hypovolemic, 64, 167
Spinal cord injury, 23, 129
Surgical ileus, 91, 189
Trisomy 21, 3, 113
Urolithiasis, 82, 179
Ventricular septal defect (VSD), 67, 169
Wound healing, 6, 116